Stroke

Overcoming My Worst Nightmare

Sara Marie Anderson

Global Touchstones

Stroke: Overcoming My Worst Nightmare

Published by:

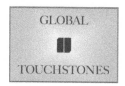

Global Touchstones

3183 Wilshire Blvd. NUM 196C29

Los Angeles, CA 90010, USA

FAX: +1 866 530 5692

http://www.globaltouchstones.com

ISBN 978-0-9909086-3-0 paperback

Typeset in Baskerville, system LyX-LaTeX 2_ε

For my extraordinary parents – Gary and Sharon Anderson

Contents

My Happy Pre-stroke Life

ON JUNE 3, 2009, I awoke to the birds chirping outside my bedroom window in Los Angeles. I was in a good place in my life. I had just moved into a beautiful home with my boyfriend at the time, Peter. We were excited about exploring the next stage of our relationship. As a language instructor at USC, I had just begun my summer vacation, so I was thinking about what to do during my time off until the next school year began in August. Would I visit friends in Hawaiii where I had lived from 2004 until 2007? Would I visit my family in Wisconsin? Would I accompany Peter to Sweden to visit his mother? Life felt truly free and full of wonderful possibilities. Little did I know on that wonderful morning that I would nearly die in the next twenty-four hours.

Peter and I had spent six months looking for just the right

house in Los Angeles. We had done a lot of research to prepare for open houses to visit on our weekends. So we were really thrilled when we found a nice home in a beautiful neighborhood. Our house was a sunny yellow ranch-style with a birch tree in the front yard. We were excited to move from our respective West Hollywood apartments into our home on April 25. A few weeks later, we were still immersed in rooms full of boxes when we both left town for ten days to visit our families for Mother's Day. I returned home to Wisconsin, while Peter went to Texas. We didn't have much time to unpack, since we had only been in our new home for three weeks. Still, I knew I would have the whole summer to unpack, or so I thought. Instead, my whole world turned upside down, when I suffered a massive stroke suddenly on June 3, 2009.

I have always believed in the importance of being positive and always tried to lead my life looking on the bright side of everything that happens. I believe this mindset, combined with my faith and the endless love provided to me by my parents, greatly helped me in my journey to recovery after my stroke. All my physical abilities were taken away that day, very unfairly, and it would have been very easy to just give up. However, I chose to accept my situation and fight hard to see how much of my abilities I could regain. "Normalcy" was my end goal, which I realize now is actually a very ambitious plan when dealing with strokes. A therapist once told me that "no one gets out of a stroke without deficits," but I was still determined to see how much I could minimize those deficits with a lot of hard work and my strong emotional dedication.

Wanting to minimize deficits was a huge goal of mine. However, spreading my story was as well. I wanted to help prevent future strokes for those other unfortunate women who as I did blindly believe their doctors, since they sometimes, unintention-ally, prescribe medications that are not compatible. I typed this entire book with only my right hand using the computer. Think of that accomplishment occasionally as you read further. Try to type an email with only one hand, and you'll quickly see how completely frustrating it becomes. I used to enjoy typing, but after the stroke I absolutely hated it because it became so difficult. So you might ask why didn't I wait to write a book until typing was easier for me? I didn't want to wait because I felt I had a cautionary but very important story to tell. I feel my stroke could have been prevented, and maybe I can save other lives or others from a tough disability by telling my story here. These thoughts compelled me to begin this book as soon as I could, as soon as possible, regardless of how frustrating I knew that task would be.

Before the stroke, I was very healthy: 5'8", 110 lbs., 27 years old. I exercised daily and I had followed a vegetarian diet for seven years. Actually, one of the first things I did in our new house was pin up my gym class schedule on the cork board in the kitchen. I highlighted the classes I had planned to attend each week. I remember not too long before the stroke, jogging down a hill at Runyon Canyon in Los Angeles and thinking I was so lucky to be healthy and not have a sprained ankle or something to prevent me from doing this running. I think this memory is very ironic because I would soon suffer an illness that in fact was going to keep me from being that active for several years, maybe even permanently.

On the morning of June 3, I ate a whole-wheat English muffin and a banana for breakfast. Then I headed to a Bodyworks class at the gym. I really liked cardio, so even after the class I would often stay on the elliptical machine for a while longer. However, that day, I went directly home, sensing a migraine beginning at the end of the class.

Actually, I had suffered from migraines for seven years and typically had one every month. However, the week or so before my stroke, I had a migraine about every other day. The frequency concerned me because it was out of the ordinary. However, when I called to schedule an appointment for a check-up, I was told there was no availability. So I packed up my gym bag with my water bottle, iPod, towel and magazine and headed home to rest. I never got to rest. Instead, I went home to begin my own worst nightmare.

Sara and Rachel hiking in Hawaii

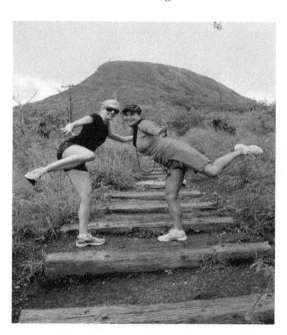

CHAPTER 1

Almost Too Late

RUSTRATING. HUMBLING. SLOW. Those three words best sum up my story of survival from having an unexpected and massive stroke at the age of twenty-seven. It's hard to believe such an event could happen to me, but sadly, the aftermath soon became all too real. Throughout my journey, many family members and friends have commented, and I agree, that you never know just how precious life is until a tragic event happens to you or a loved one. Despite the odds, however, I am fortunate to know the value of life. Why? I survived even though my path of recovery continued for many years—frustrating, humbling and incredibly slow.

My initial prescription for birth control pills began when I was seventeen due to my irregular periods. My periods were coming too often, like every other week. I may not have minded it so much if it had come once every six months, but every other week was a lot of blood to lose. Honestly, what woman would be okay with her period showing up every other week? So my mother took me to a gynecologist for a physical and I was put on birth control pills to regulate my cycles. I did not suffer any side effects from the medication, so I stayed on them because they did help.

Very little is known about migraines. Doctors don't completely know why they occur or how best to treat them. What works for one individual may not work for another. For the most part, I was told that the best remedy was to take medication, close my eyes, and do my best to sleep it off. Often, my migraine would be gone by morning. I thought that was enough.

I was sitting in my political science class as an undergraduate at the University of Wisconsin-Madison when I had the visual aura for the first time. I had no idea what it was and I became very scared. Because I was so scared, I went to see a doctor shortly after the incident. The doctor diagnosed me with "just migraines." No one in my family had ever had migraines, so I didn't understand why I was getting them. I thought maybe I had a brain tumor or something more immediately severe. For me, the aura was even worse than the headache itself because losing my sense of vision and focus was so scary that I felt powerless. Sometimes when I noticed the aura coming on, I would try to ignore it and hope it would simply go away, but it never did. There was no denying it or making the aura or subsequent migraine go away.

I began to have migraine headaches with aura when I was twenty. My aura would often be triggered by looking at something bright, for example, a light reflecting off metal or a bright lamp in a dimly lit restaurant, or just the sun. As a result, I always wore sunglasses outside and was very aware of the lights around me. My auras would normally happen once a month. Sometimes, when I looked at something too bright, my vision would feel shaky at the corner of one of my eyes. The sensation was like looking at something bright, then looking away, and still seeing the after-image. This shaky after-image would then last for thirty minutes until a headache ensued. As my aura and migraine developed further, I would typically take my prescribed migraine medicine and prepare emotionally as best as I could. Thankfully, I was never working or driving when I got a migraine. Instead, I would often be at home when the migraine began, which was fortunate. It's important to note here as well that my birth control alone was not the problem. The (most likely) problem was that I was taking a combination of estrogen and progesterone as birth control while also suffering from migraines with aura.

Here's what I learned from my neurologist about the Pill since my stroke:

1. If you do not get migraines and are not on any contra-indicated medications, it is very rare for a women to suffer a stroke from hormonal birth control.

2. If you get migraines, you should *NOT* be on any hormonal medication, especially hormonal birth control that is combined with estrogen and progesterone, as it increases the risk.

3. If you experience migraines with aura, this condition greatly increases your risk for a stroke, and you absolutely should *NOT* be on hormonal birth control with a combination of estrogen and progesterone. In my mind, I now visualize blinking red lights flashing *STOP!* as an important warning to immediately discontinue any birth control that isn't progesterone only.

4. The "safer" form of birth control is progesterone-only; the

most dangerous kind is a combined progesterone and estrogen birth control. So fortunately you don't need to discontinue the Pill or hormones, just simply switch to a progesterone-only version.

5. While my only experience with taking hormones is birth control, this same warning applies to people of all ages who experience migraines with aura and take hormones for any other purpose. These people should also imagine the flashings *STOP!* warning and switch hormones to progesterone-only hormones.

A very trusted neurologist, who is also a stroke expert in Los Angeles, gave me this information. He unfortunately has had to deal with the reality of stroke in women constantly when they and their doctors don't follow these recommendations. He also informed me that this information is not that well-known among most doctors, so keep that in mind when you talk to your own. I now hope everyone will have this information and take it seriously.

While I have friends who have found a medicine that totally takes their migraine away, I never had that kind of luck. Upon experiencing the aura a few times, I learned to sense what was coming next and know that there was little I could do to prevent that aura and the migraine from running its course. From the little literature I read on the subject, everything said migraines are permanent. Yet I didn't want to feel like they were controlling my life. That said, I rarely complained to my boyfriend about my migraines and I would still go out and be social if we had plans, even if I didn't feel great. It was never easy, but I wanted to be in control of the migraines rather than having the migraines in control of me.

It's interesting to note as well that my migraines have nearly disappeared since the stroke. The neurologist who took care of me after the stroke said that having migraines with an aura should have been enough of a warning for a physician never to have prescribed the birth control pill prescribed for me. Let that speak loudly to all women in similar situations.

The main purpose of my book is to bring more awareness of the dangers of combining hormonal birth control with migraines and encourage young women to get off that medication, or at the very least have an informed conversation with their gynecologist or neurologist and switch to a much "safer," progesterone-only form of birth control.

It seemed like everyone takes the Pill these days, so I never thought that there was anything dangerous about it. I also didn't mind the added "benefits." My skin was clearer (although my skin was clear anyway with only the occasional pimple). The Pill is also supposed to protect against certain cancers, so obviously I liked that idea too. When I moved to California, a doctor changed my prescription to Yasmin, a lower hormone alternative compared to other oral contraceptive pills. That appealed to me because I liked taking less medication. It sounded safer. However, Yasmin is actually the dangerous combined estrogen and progesterone birth control medication, and because I experienced migraines with aura, I was unknowingly swallowing ticking time bombs every day.

At my last gynecology check-up before the stroke, I had discussed going off Yasmin because I had been on it for ten years and I believed it was time to give my body a break. Plus, I was curious to see if my cycle was now regulated. Additionally, I was always conscious of everything I ate and the medications I took, and thus, I was starting to question if I should even continue with the Pill at all. But my doctor assured me it was fine and told me not to worry. My migraines continued, so I consulted another doctor about them. That doctor, from the same clinic, prescribed Midrin to help control my headaches. I should point out here that this clinic used electronic records, so all the doctors I saw were well aware of my medical history and which medications I had been prescribed. Migraine medication and hormonal birth control are contra-indicated treatments. I have since learned that the bigger contra-indication is taking combined estrogen and progesterone birth control when you experience migraines with aura. That was most likely the cause of my stroke. Fortunately, progesterone-only forms of birth control are "safer," so all young women: please do talk to your doctors about switching to a progesterone-only form of birth control medication.

In reading my favorite magazines that target young women, I often see Q&As that address the Pill. They always seem to favor taking the Pill and say it is one of the most reliable forms of birth control. It breaks my heart that the other side of the story on this important issue, i.e., those who have suffered major medical issues as a result of taking the Pill, are never asked to express their side. Perhaps this is because the risk is small, so the editors don't want to scare their readers. However, I am living proof that the risk is truly there, and I certainly believe that this side of the story should be heard, especially when one can easily switch to a progesterone-only birth control rather than simply stopping birth control entirely. If my story makes women think twice about their birth control, learn more about how it can potentially affect the female body and make the best decisions for themselves using that information, then my stroke will have another very positive outcome for the future.

If I could turn back the clock, obviously there is no way I would have taken the Pill with combined estrogen and progesterone because I would have known about the potential dangers. However, it is important to note here that I am not against the Pill. Rather, I am a "know-all-your-risks" example of the dangers of taking hormonal birth control. To repeat, progesterone-only birth control is the safest pill to take, and I definitely want young women to know their risks and take the safest kind of birth control.

Every time I had an appointment at the hospital, I was always asked what medications I was on and I always replied "Yasmin and Midrin." Always. They were also aware of the fact that I experienced migraines with aura. The hospital's electronic records clearly show those medications, and my Ob/GYN, my General Practitioner, pharmacist, and even the computer failed to make the connection that those medications carry contradictory warnings. All these venues failed to bring this to my attention. They failed to alert me to the danger of taking combined estrogen and progesterone birth control while suffering from migraines with aura.

Of course you trust your doctor to know which medications are safe and which medications interact with each other. You would also think that a warning would pop up on their computer screens, so doctors would know to alert their patients. I strongly believe that every person has a right to know if they're taking contra-indicated medication even if the possibility of a tragedy is small. No health warning should ever be ignored or swept under the rug due to a medical provider's decision. It is our right as patients to know when we are prescribed contra-indicated medications, so we can decide if we want to continue taking them or not. I want to see a change made so that it actually becomes the law for doctors to alert patients whenever a patient is on contra-indicated medications. It is simply not ethical medical practice for the doctor alone to make that call. However, I also believe that it is the patient's responsibility to read a medication's warnings and contra-indications themselves before taking a medication. I advise everyone to do this for ANY medication. Even a simple internet search for the medication's reviews will give you some questions to ask your doctor.

The week before my stroke, I had so many migraines, about one every other day that I ran out of Midrin. My migraines were obviously out of control, so I called for an appointment to see a migraine specialist. I was told I first needed a referral, which would take a few days, and only then could an appointment be booked per availability. In the meantime, I needed more migraine medication, so I ordered more Midrin and more Yasmin over the phone. Despite the fact that both medicines carry warnings about using the other at the same time, the medications were delivered a few days later, ironically even together in the same package and even more tragically, on the same day of my stroke. My mother urged me right before the stroke to go to the doctor and just sit in the office until someone would see me. However, I believed I could wait a little longer for a scheduled appointment. I didn't want to be pushy, but looking back now, I should have listened and I should have been very pushy. Yes, Mom, you were right and I should have listened to you. Thus, there were two contra-indications in my case:

1. Taking the birth control pill and migraine medication concurrently.

2. Suffering from migraines with aura and taking a prescription for combined estrogen and progesterone hormonal birth control. I've since learned that the latter is more likely the cause of my stroke.

It would have been safer if I had been on a progesterone-only form of birth control even when I was having migraines with aura.

My dad at my bedside a few days after my stroke

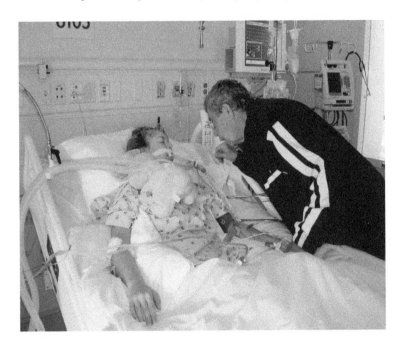

CHAPTER 2

The Emergency Continues

O N THE DAY of my stroke, I had gone to the gym. I was starting to take classes there: Pilates and Bodyworks Plus Abs, which is a mixture of cardio and dumbbells. Bodyworks Plus Abs was the class I attended right before my stroke. I actually hated lifting weights and doing strength training, but I thought I would do it more regularly if I attended this class. I enjoyed cardio more. My standard workout consisted of sixty minutes on the elliptical machine, but I knew that six minutes of cardio is a lot on any machine. Even ten minutes feels like a lot on the elliptical, so I was definitely getting a real workout! I usually did my elliptical routine about four to five days a week. Then Peter and I would hike on the weekends.

I was physically fit.

When I returned home from the gym that day, I noticed a delivery truck at the house. We were getting new furniture. "Hi Peter," I said.

"Hey Sara. The furniture guys just showed up with the delivery. How was the gym today?"

"Okay, although I'm getting another migraine. I'm going to take a shower and lie down for a bit."

I went in the bathroom to take that shower, entered the shower, but suddenly I felt too light-headed to continue with it. So I got out of the shower, put on my robe, and sat down on the dark blue bathroom rug in front of the sink. I called out to Peter who was in the living room.

"Peter?!" Peter quickly came to the door, looked in, and saw me sitting on the ground right below the sink. My hands were gripping my head.

"Sara, what's wrong?"

"I'm having a visual aura. I think it was triggered by the fluorescent lights at the gym. I can feel a migraine coming on."

Peter wasn't used to living with me, so he didn't really know how often I got migraines, but he knew I had had several that past week.

"Sara, what can I do?" he asked.

"I don't know. My tongue feels numb!"

"Did you take your medicine?"

"No, not even my vitamins yet! I just want to lie down."

I now remember hoping that he wouldn't need the information about my medicine.

According to Peter, I had started to hyperventilate. I also felt the numbness spreading from my mouth to my tongue and cheeks.

Of course if either of us then had been at all aware of even basic stroke information, we would've realized that facial numbness is one of the main symptoms of a stroke and called 911.

In its 9 July 2018 *Journal*, the American Heart Association strongly advised heeding the acronym *BE-FAST* to Remember the Warning Signs of a Stroke: BE-FAST (Balance, Eyes, Face, Arm, Speech, Time)! If you notice changes in any of these areas, call 911 immediately!

At first I only noticed facial numbness, although after my stroke, balance, eyes and arms were also an issue. Time is so critical. If you notice anything even slightly suspicious, like slurred speech, dial 911 immediately! Better to be safe than sorry! I walked over to the bed to lie down. I put the pillows under my feet to keep my feet elevated. I had heard somewhere that you should do that if you not feeling your best.

"Do you want to go see a doctor right now?" he asked me.

"Maybe." I knew, however, we would most likely have to wait without having an appointment, so this initially dissuaded me from going. Still, it felt weird with the numbness in my mouth, and since I had been having so many migraines recently, I thought it would be a good idea to see a doctor. Normally, when I had a migraine I would turn off the lights and lie down for a bit and hope I felt better when I got up again. However, it was still early, before noon, so I couldn't go to sleep for the day. I didn't take naps.

Peter asked now if he should call an ambulance. Of course not—*It's just a migraine!* I had never been in an ambulance, and I certainly wasn't going to make this situation the first time—not for just a migraine. Peter doubted if an ambulance would even come for a twenty-seven-year-old woman who was complaining of a migraine. On a side note, know that they will come, and you should call if you're ever experiencing a strange symptom medically. So, he first called the hospital number on the medical health card in my wallet to see if there was a closer location. He could drive me there. The hospital was only five to six miles away, but with LA traffic you never could be sure how long it would take to get there.

I got into Peter's car without problem. I thought I was just going to get a quick check-up. I never thought I wouldn't be seeing the home I had just moved into with Peter for the next six months! In the car, I immediately put on my dark sunglasses due to severe sensitivity to light, and I reclined Peter's passenger seat as much as possible to lie down. I kept the sunglasses on even in the hospital. As always, my sensitivity to light was extremely heightened during a migraine.

About halfway to the hospital, I asked, "Peter, could you pull over? I think I'm going to throw up." Peter pulled over, and I opened the door and threw up. I didn't think anything about it because I had heard about people who were having migraines becoming nauseated and throwing up. But I had never vomited before when I was having a migraine.

We pulled up to "Urgent Care" (the ER) and waited for a ridiculous 4.5 hours before we got a room! Outrageous! That was probably an emergency waiting room record. Once I was in the private ER room, looking back now, I realize that precious time was lost in evaluating my condition and administrating the serious care I needed. That negligence only continued to escalate.

I had signed in when we first got to the ER. Then I got into a wheelchair, unaware that I would have to work very hard to get out of that wheelchair in the months to come. I also got a vomit bag at the front desk because I was still occasionally vomiting, even though I had nothing left in my stomach to throw up, so I was just dry heaving. Gross, I know. Peter and I sat, and we waited, and waited, and waited. We waited longer and longer in the waiting room. I just wanted to lie down. The staff said all the beds were currently being used, so there was no bed for me. They finally took my vital signs at the front desk, checked my temperature and blood pressure and then escorted me back to the waiting room to continue the wait. Calling 911 is definitely the way to go in an emergency; it was foolish of Peter and me not to have done this.

I felt very warm, so I insisted they check my blood pressure and temperature again, as I was sure both were high. Both came back as normal. We were both surprised, as Peter remembers that I felt warm then. In the waiting room, I remember sitting in the wheelchair and thinking, so this is what it feels like to die? Of course I thought I was being over-dramatic, but ironically I was thinking right on target. I also remember wondering how to make the hospital staff believe that my situation was urgent and that I needed to be seen immediately. Obviously being in "urgent-care" in a wheelchair, wearing dark sunglasses and vomiting into a bag were not throwing out any red flags to anyone there at the time.

"Peter, I'm starting to feel better now, so could we go home so I can lie down?" I asked him that because it was taking so long to get treatment, and I just wanted to rest. I didn't really feel any better, but I thought anything had to be better than sitting there in that waiting room.

"I think it's just another migraine," I told him. "I just want to go home and lie down and rest." I was trying hard to justify my desire to go home.

Peter and I were both getting anxious. I now wondered if an ambulance would have been faster in the end, as then we probably would have at least seen a doctor more quickly or been given a bed where I could lie down. Again, yes, we definitely should have called 911. Apparently, I had drawn an incredibly unlucky day to have to come into such a crowded waiting room. Finally, after 4.5 hours of waiting, my name was called. I was so happy that my way-too-long wait for treatment was finally over.

The doctor asked me what was going on. I explained I had suffered from migraines for about seven years and almost always experienced the visual aura with each migraine. In fact, the aura was how I distinguished migraines from other headaches. I also told him that I had been at the gym earlier that day, and it's possible that the large fluorescent lights there might have triggered my migraine. Yet this migraine felt different. I was experiencing facial numbness and vomiting as well, and both of these symptoms were really unusual for me. Despite the fact that facial numbness is one of the most common stroke symptoms, this staff diagnosed me with only having a "severe migraine," and they started a nausea drip, a rehydration drip and a morphine drip for the pain and to put me to sleep. That was the worst treatment they could have done. They didn't even consider a stroke because of my age, but I believe it was their job that day to consider ALL possibilities. They failed miserably. They didn't do their job during my initial hospital stay and with obvious stroke symptoms they didn't even contact a neurologist.

Strokes don't discriminate by age. In my rehab experience later on, I met a mother whose toddler son had actually had a stroke at age two! I've even heard of strokes happening in the womb! People assume that most strokes happen to the elderly, but strokes do happen with younger people, and my doctors and/or triage nurse should have recognized that fact, especially when I said that this migraine felt "different."

Since I was knocked unconscious by the morphine for a couple of hours, the doctors could not tell I was actually undergoing a deadly stroke that was depleting the oxygen to my brain. The problem became apparent only when I was supposed to wake up, but I didn't. The medical staff then thought maybe I was a "lightweight" on morphine, so they only gave me more time to wake up.

"Sara!" They shouted at me after another hour, but still no response came from me. They felt that was odd, but they continued to think I was only having an "idiocentric reaction" to the morphine and needed more time to sleep the drug off. The doctors did not seem overly concerned at all. I only needed more time to come around properly.

The doctors gave me the drug Narcan to try to reverse the morphine, but still nothing happened. They opened my eyelids and saw that my pupils were fixed and dilated. It was then they finally decided to give me a CT scan, but still, the head ER doctor, who wasn't a neurologist, didn't notice anything abnormal on the scan. She didn't even forward my scan to a neurologist to read. Then they gave me a spinal tap, and that came back clean too. I later learned that the spinal tap probably made my stroke more severe and should never have been performed. I was told to imagine a garden hose turned on but with a kink, and then removing the kink and the pressure releasing. Then, they drew some blood to test, and just gave me more time to wake up, figuring I would eventually do so.

After a second round of Narcan, I still did not wake up. The head ER doctor finally decided to send my CT-scan to a neurologist to read. After looking at it, the neurologist sent the scan to a remote location for more analysis. Their concern was really mounting now. At 4 a.m., that same neurologist at the remote location finally saw the blood clot that was killing me and told them to rush me to a different location where they were better equipped to treat a stroke. They rushed me to a new location in an ambulance, and this was the location where they saved my life. I feel the need to emphasize how remarkable this second location of the same medical center was to me. It was night and day. While the first location really dropped the ball and made many critical medical mistakes that almost killed me, the second location did everything flawlessly to keep me alive and ultimately saved my life. Remember, I had avoided taking an ambulance earlier because it seemed silly to call an ambulance for a migraine. A lot of precious time was lost before I was finally diagnosed correctly. It was now fourteen hours since I had arrived at the hospital and nine hours since being put under with morphine.

Time is critical in all strokes. In fact, since my stroke, we have seen "TIME IS BRAIN" warnings about stroke symptoms in multiple medical locations. Unfortunately, I was robbed of that critical time due to the negligence of the medical staff that was treating me at the time. I realize now how incredibly accurate and important the "TIME IS BRAIN" warning is for all of us.

At the hospital, they immediately put me in an MRA machine to look at my brain further. They saw that a blood clot was blocking oxygen from entering my brain and had thus caused the stroke. My stroke was massive and I had been stroking for fourteen hours. I was close to death.

Shortly thereafter, the chief surgeon came into the waiting room and motioned for Peter. Peter and I were not married. The surgeon said that he needed to talk to a parent to get authorization for medical care since I was unconscious. He found my sister Lisa's number in my phone and called her, and Lisa immediately called my mom.

CHAPTER 3

In the ER, the Emergency Still Continues

HE SURGEONS HAD to remove the blood clot, or I would surely die. Had they diagnosed me correctly as having a stroke earlier, per all the multiple signs that were clearly present, they could have given me a clot-busting drug to break up the clot, thereby avoiding my life or death surgery and saving a lot of my brain from dying. However, they diagnosed me way too late, ridiculously late, and almost too late. I was later told I was lucky to be alive because the stroke had been so massive. That stroke also very unfortunately affected both sides of my body, as it occurred in a complicated area of my brainstem, in the basilar artery, so it severely affected my balance, coordination, speech, vision and motor skills, leaving greater overall weakness on my left side than my right, although the right side was also affected. However, I'm still very grateful the stroke didn't affect my memory or language (although it did take months before I could make any sounds and eventually speak). I don't know what I would have done if I couldn't remember my family or friends. How awful that would have been!

CHAPTER **4**

My Living Guardian Angels (my parents)

I WOULD LIKE to acknowledge some of the key people who constantly stayed by my side, beginning with my exceptional parents. I have the best parents in the world. My parents are divorced, but they are the only divorced parents I know of that are still close friends. I mean, they really ARE friends. Secondly, my parents left everything to be with me and take care of me from day one of my stroke. My dad is a retired teacher, and he gave up all of his activities to be with me. My mom, not yet retired then was a rural mail carrier in LaCrosse, Wisconsin, and she missed six months of work to come to be with me. They both also have their own lives and friends, and they left all of them to be with me. They sacrificed greatly, and for that loving care, I will always be hugely grateful. I can't imagine

Stroke

what it must have been like for them, so I want to try to tell their personal story here in my own words.

CHAPTER 5

My Family's Nightmare Begins

MY MOM AWOKE June 4 to the phone ringing. She looked at the caller ID and saw it was my sister, Lisa. She was immediately worried because it was such an early hour for a call, around 6 a.m.

"Lisa, are you okay? Why are you calling so early?" she anxiously asked.

"I'm okay, but you need to call Peter. He just called me and told me Sara has had a stroke!"

"What are you talking about?!! I'll call him right away."

Then my mom called Peter.

"Peter, it's Sharon, Sara's Mom. I just got a frantic call from Lisa. She told me Sara has had a stroke and I needed to call you immediately!"

"Yes, it's true. Sara went to the hospital for a migraine, but now they have determined it's a stroke! The doctors need your permission to operate and remove a blood clot from the back of her brain. I am going to put you on the phone with the head doctor right now, as time is critical."

"Okay," my incredibly nervous mother responded.

"Sharon, this is Dr. Feng. I need your verbal approval to operate on Sara and remove the blood clot still in her brainstem. It is a life and death situation, so we need to move very quickly."

"What about a clot-busting drug? Can't you give her that?" He then added "I would strongly encourage you and her family to come to California, as I can't guarantee she'll still be alive when you get here. We are well beyond the window of time for administering that drug."

Now my mom worries about everything anyway, even more than most moms do, so you can imagine how she felt hearing a doctor say he didn't know if I would be alive when she got to me. Any mother would be frantic, but my mother, who worries if I don't return her calls within twenty-four hours even when she tells me not to call her back, was absolutely terrified.

"Dr. Feng, are you even a very good doctor?"

"I like to think that I am."

She gave him her permission to operate on my brain to try to save my life.

My mom then spoke with Peter further. As a devout Catholic, she was adamant that he ask for a priest to read me the *Sacrament of the Sick*—also known as the *Last Rites*. He had his brother make the arrangements, and a priest promptly came into my hospital room pre-operation to give me the *Sacrament of the Sick*. My mom was very relieved to hear about that later that same day. After hanging up with Peter and the doctor, my mom called my dad, Gary. Dad was getting ready to head out to the golf course. His plans, of course, immediately changed.

"Gary, Sara's had a stroke. We need to go to California immediately!"

"What?!"

"I know it's awful and sudden. Peter called Lisa, and she called me. I've already spoken to the doctor and we have to leave immediately!"

"Okay, I'll start packing."

While my Dad packed for the unexpected trip, my mom called my sister and told her to start packing for California too. Then she called my brother, Brian, in Winona, Minnesota, and then, her own parents, and her friend Elna (she would have to watch her cat). My sister called some of my best friends in Wisconsin because she had their cell phone numbers. All were totally shocked to hear the news because I was so young and presumably very healthy. My mom then went into protective mother mode. When she gets into this mode she is stronger than anyone I've known. She was able to keep everyone in a positive state of mind, in spite of the terror around them. She contacted Delta in Minneapolis, explained the emergency and bought eight tickets for the noon flight.

Everyone—my mom, Dad, sister Lisa and her three kids (Tyler, Tanner and Isabella), my brother Brian and his and my sister-in-law Melanie, were going to meet in LaCrosse, Wisconsin. My mom was getting radiation for breast cancer treatments at the time, and she left first for LaCrosse. She called and scheduled an emergency radiation treatment for herself. She also had to get her surgical arm wrapped tightly because changes in air pressure on the plane could cause a condition known as Lymphedema (swelling in the arm near the surgical incision). On the way to the Cancer Center, she called our priest, Father Cook in Viroqua, Wisconsin, and told him what had happened. He was in disbelief, but told her that he was on his way to morning Mass, and he would say Mass for me.

On a positive note, my mom beat breast cancer. On April 1, 2009, she had her annual mammogram and they found a very tiny piece of breast cancer. It was fortunately very early and barely visible, just at Stage One. In fact, my mom was late in scheduling her annual mammogram that year, so she felt guilty after receiving those results. The cancer was so tiny that the doctor reassured her, saying it could have been undetectable if she had had the mammogram a few months earlier. On April 15 they did a lumpectomy and she received radiation treatment rather than chemotherapy. She was supposed to receive radiation from May until July that year, but she ended up being in California with me most of that time, so she didn't receive nearly the amount of radiation treatment she would have had if she could have remained in Wisconsin. Despite everything, she has remained cancer-free. I am very thankful for that.

Father Cook also notified our church's prayer circle. The health clinic nurse who assisted my mom with the radiation treatment also asked if she could take my name to the Franciscan Sisters of Perpetual Adoration. The Sisters pray in shifts twenty-four hours a day. Everyone at the health clinic said they would be praying as well. As word of my condition spread like wildfire, I learned later that I was included in prayer groups that circled the globe. I am very grateful to have received so many prayers going into surgery and throughout my recovery. My mom says that God reached out and held me in the palm of His hand during this awful time.

Once all of my family was together in LaCrosse, they squeezed into two cars and drove the three hours to the Minneapolis airport. The plane tickets were waiting, and they were easily cleared for the flight. Only my brother, Brian, and his wife, Melanie, had visited me in LA before the stroke. My two nephews and niece had never even been in a plane. Tyler was eight, Tanner was five, and Isabella was three. My sister absolutely hates flying, but my condition was so serious it was preoccupying everyone's thoughts. On the way to the airport, Peter's brother, Adam, called and told my mom that I had survived the clot removal surgery. He also asked how many people in my family were flying to be with me so he could arrange transportation for them to the hospital once they arrived.

My mom has always had a strange intuition. I remember when I was about ten, she was taking my friend and me to ski school in LaCrosse, Wisconsin. My sister, Lisa, was late coming home, so my mother was monitoring the oncoming traffic to see if we could meet her. We started driving down a hill. You couldn't see the bottom because the road curved. Yet Mom started freaking out and saying Lisa's name. As we turned the corner, we saw an ambulance and my sister Lisa's car (she had been in a car accident). Fortunately, Lisa was okay because she was wearing her seatbelt. I only bring it up here because that was the first time that I witnessed my mom's intuition firsthand. Later on, I would often call my mom before a flight and ask her, "Do you have any bad feelings about this flight?" She would always tell me, "No." Like my sister, I am a nervous flyer, but I didn't inherit my mom's intuition. Even before and during the stroke, nothing inside me was saying, "This is going to be a bad day for you," or, "Go straight to the hospital." My mom, on the other hand, had been waking up at around 4 a.m. for a couple of months prior to my stroke with an ominous feeling. She had urged me earlier to go to the clinic and wait there until they would see me for my concerning migraines but I decided instead to just wait for an appointment that never came.

On the flight to California, my mom said she had been praying non-stop since the morning phone call. Then suddenly she had a very calm feeling as though a voice had spoken to her. She knew from that moment that I would be okay, not just alive, but totally okay. I remembered hearing her say this, and I believed her words during my recovery. I often asked her about it because I trusted her and her intuition. She said she had just looked at my dad on the flight and said, "She's going to be okay." He asked, "How do you know?" She said, "I just know." She told my sister, my brother and his wife. They just looked at her in surprise but didn't question her. She never told my dad until much later that the doctor had told her my life was in jeopardy or that I may not be alive when they got to LA. I guess this decision was a good one, as it was one less thing for him to worry about. Given how much my mom worries, I thought it was a great sign that she had a very calm feeling during this anxious situation.

I occasionally still ask her to retell it to me even now, years later, because I believe it was a sign from God that everything was going to be okay. During the flight, my family discussed the nature of strokes. Their knowledge was very limited because thankfully, no one in my family had ever suffered a stroke before. This lack of knowledge was a blessing in disguise as well because everyone believed that I would recover completely and quickly. My sister-in-law's father, Tom, had suffered a stroke when he was fifty-five. The doctors told him he'd never walk again, but he did. He even walked Melanie down the aisle at her wedding.

I may have been the most ignorant of all of us about strokes. Before the stroke I knew a stroke was 1. A medical condition. 2. Very bad. 3. You never wanted to have one. 4. It typically affects one side of your body. That's it! That's all I knew. Pretty limited, but why should I know more? I certainly wasn't at risk for having one. I was young and healthy with no family history of stroke! So I didn't even know how to appropriately consider stroke as a warning side effect of the Pill. When my family got to LA, they were surprised to see a driver holding a sign that said, "Anderson." The van Adam had arranged for them was waiting, and they came straight to the hospital.

Inside the ICU, I simply lay motionless hooked up to many machines. Fortunately, I survived the first surgery and the stroke. The doctor later told Peter that only 25 percent of basilar artery stroke victims even survive the stroke, and recovery is always the most difficult. Still, my young age and my physical fitness were strong allies for recovery. Even so, the doctor repeated once again that the first three days after a stroke are very dangerous for all stroke patients. Shortly thereafter, my family arrived. Peter's family was already at the hospital.

"Where's Sara?!" My mom anxiously asked.

"She's in the far room down the hall. Unconscious. The doctor says she will be closely monitored here in the ICU under twenty-four-hour observation. They feel they are still in the stage of trying to save her life," Peter said.

"What else?!"

"It's too early to know details about any damages, but the stroke was massive, and it hit at a critical area in her brainstem."

Dr. Feng met my parents upon arrival and told them "We were able to successfully remove the blood clot from her brain, but she will need twenty-four-hour supervision for the next few days in the ICU. She's alive, but the first three days are very dangerous with strokes. Sara's had a very serious brain injury, and we don't know yet what exactly has been damaged. She is not out of the woods. Things are still very serious for how her brain will respond to the major surgery. She's in critical condition."

"But at least she's alive!" My mom then ran in to see me. A couple of weeks into my ER stay, the hospital had considered that maybe the blood clot had formed because there was a hole in my heart or my lungs. However, upon examining those organs they found no evidence of that situation.

When my family arrived at the hospital, I was in a sleep-like state, almost like a coma. The doctors were astounded to see how many people had traveled immediately all the way from Wisconsin. I was unaware of anything at the time but I wasn't surprised at all to hear about it later because I know how amazing my family is. I have no memory of the first week in the ICU. My mom came into the hospital room, which was always freezing cold to preserve my body temperature so my brain wouldn't swell, and she just grabbed my hand and said, "Sara, it's Mom." While I was in this coma-like state, I could not open my eyes, talk, or move, but I could hear her. She later told me I cried when she was holding my hand and talking to me. She explained that I was very, very sick, and I should not fight the tubes and wires. She told me to relax and rest, so I would get better. My dad, brother and sister also came to visit and then everyone settled into the waiting room to live out the next five days. They stayed with Peter at night, but my mom stayed with me in the hospital.

Per hospital policy, my nephews and niece were not allowed to come in and see me in the ICU because they were too young.

On the last day of their visit, after days of being very patient, my mom told the nurse that they needed to see me because they needed to understand why they had taken the flight to see their Aunt Sara. One time when the nurse was rolling me down the hall for one of my many cat-scans, the kids walked to the nearby hallway to see my bed go by, and Tyler, the oldest at age eight, yelled "Hi Sara!" The nurse said I reacted, so I must have heard him. Any reaction to stimulus also meant that I was still "there." It was a very positive sign.

Dr. Navdeep Sangha, a neurologist, watched over me and remained with my case throughout my month-long stay in the ICU. My parents adored him because he was the only one who sat and talked with them through everything and answered all their many questions. You can imagine how terrified and confused everyone was. He was also surprised to see all the many visitors who had flown so far to be with me.

"Dr. Sangha, what should we expect next?", my mom asked.

"Well, young people have a lot of brain mass in their heads, so we'll probably need to remove a bone from the rear of her skull to allow space for her brain to swell," he explained.

"That sounds very risky!"

"It is, but it's not as risky as not performing it."

"What would happen if you didn't do that?"

"The brain would probably swell downwards into her spinal cord and permanently paralyze her."

The procedure was dangerous, but not performing the surgery would be even more dangerous. That night, my mom stayed with me in the ER, resting on a tiny cot in my freezing room, praying for me and watching over me.

Sure enough, early the next day, as Dr. Sangha predicted,

the doctors said they needed to perform a second surgery. They needed to remove a bone from the rear of my skull to make enough room for my brain to swell. The doctors approached my mom to have her sign the permission slip to do the surgery. She was alone with me at the hospital, so it took a lot of strength for her to give permission for the second time for doctors to operate on her child's brain. The hospital chaplain came and sat with her until the rest of the family arrived.

Later, my sister told me that her head hurt a lot before and during the surgery, and then her headache went away. She attributes this reaction to a sort of sisterly bond and took it as a sign that I was okay even before the doctors gave my family any news. Sure enough, the doctors reported that my surgery went well, but still to understand that I was in the midst of a critical period, as my brain began its initial recovery from these significant surgeries. My mom never doubted that I would be okay, based on the calm feeling she had had on the plane trip from Wisconsin. She said it would have been much worse if she had not known in her heart that I was going to be okay, and she hated it whenever the doctors weren't as optimistic as she was.

After a long day in the ICU, the doctors told everyone to go get something to eat because everything seemed stable. They went to Shakey's Pizza around the corner. However, before they even finished dinner, my mom got a call from another doctor who told her the pressure in my brain was increasing, and he needed to operate immediately to put a drain tube into the top of my head. My mom made another difficult decision and approved my third cranial surgery in two days! This surgery would be at the front of my skull to remove the excess water on my brain that had collected there from the swelling. They were basically going to drill into my brain to drain the liquid and insert a tap, so they could drain it as needed over the next several days.

Everyone hustled back to the ER again and paced in the waiting room until I came out of that surgery. This was another risky procedure, but I was able to get through it. It was a big relief for everyone. It left me with a tube sticking out of my head, and they constantly put a level on it to keep the appropriate pressure level on my brain. At the end of the day, all the family left the waiting room at visitor closing time. But once again, my mom stayed in my freezing ER room overnight on a small cot, watching over me.

When the doctors removed bone in the front and back of my head, they also shaved those parts of my head, and it took a LONG time for that hair to grow back! The back of my head where it was shaved wasn't so bad because you couldn't see it; however, the front looked really stupid while it was growing out. It looked like I had bangs, but only half bangs on one side of my head. It seemed to take forever for those patches of bangs to grow to a decent length. Rightfully so, however, the doctors were only thinking about saving my life at the time, not how my hair would look in the months to come, but I had to live with it all growing out which definitely sucked. I know this reaction may seem vain and quite silly in the grand scheme of all that had happened to me, but it's a woman thing. Women know how long it takes hair to grow. Men probably don't understand it as much. But yes, it is a funny side note to remember and one detail that we can smile about now, knowing the severity of the situation at the time. Really, I was lucky that they didn't shave my entire head! I thank whoever it was who was an advocate for me to keep most of my hair. I later discovered that it was my mom. To this day I still have a divot at the front of my head where they removed the bone to drain the excess water on my brain from the swelling. You can feel the divot, but fortunately, you cannot see it, as my hair has grown enough to cover it.

While waiting for me to be brought back to my ICU room, one of the doctors came and handed my mom a brown bag with my name on it. She asked what was in the bag. The doctor told her it was the hair they had shaved from the back of my head. She felt weak and even nauseous. She took the bag and put it in her suitcase in my room. She still has the bag to this day, but she has never opened it.

So I had survived three brain surgeries, but I was still not cleared by the doctors as being out of the danger zone. All through that week, my family stayed in the waiting room all day and night, from 8 a.m.–11 p.m., waiting on any doctor's updates and taking turns, two at a time, to sit at my bedside.

Eventually, my mom, Brian, Melanie, Lisa and the kids had to return to Wisconsin. My mom had to get back to her radiation treatments, and Brian, Lisa, and Melanie had to get back to their jobs. It was hard for them to leave me, virtually lifeless and connected to a wall of machines. On the day they left, my mom sat at my bedside and talked to me for a long time. She explained she had to leave for a week or two to finish her radiation treatment but she promised she would be back soon. Somehow, I knew that she would. Then suddenly, I opened a small sliver of one eye. My brother and Melanie were in the room at the time. My mom quickly sent Melanie to alert everyone in the waiting room. I don't remember this event, but I have been told that everyone came rushing into my ER room with lots of tears and big smiles of hope. Everyone talked to me as I looked up at them with one half of an eye. My family was all there, closely huddled around me. The nurse even let the kids come in to see me before they had to leave. My nephew, Tanner, just said, "Sara's sick. She can't wake up."

Before my mom returned home for medical treatment, she remembered something she knew was important to bring to the ER, when the doctors worked to save my life. She then made sure my stuffed rabbit, Connie, came to be with me at the hospital.

Connie is the stuffed rabbit I received from the Easter Bunny when I was four years old. She has traveled with me everywhere. She came with me to Spain when I moved there as an undergraduate to improve my Spanish language skills. She also moved with me to Honolulu when I got my master's degree and to Los Angeles where I was living at the time of the stroke. Unfortunately, she now had to live with me in the hospital. My family was very familiar with Connie and her role in my life. The nurses also got to know Connie, and when my parents had to leave the room, the nurses would put my arm around Connie. I have a vague memory of this experience. Even when a person is unconscious, I have learned it's important to treat them as if they are awake and understanding because no one knows if and how much they're actually hearing you. The nurses also asked my mom to make charts with the names of my family and friends. They also asked her to write down where I had lived so they could talk about these places with me. Although I was unconscious, my brain was not turned off.

After my family had to leave, my dad moved into my freezing ER room and spent every night on the tiny cot nearby. Every hour on the hour, the nurses would come in to read my vitals and take blood. My dad says bells and whistles went off all through the night, as the machines monitored my breathing and pumped me full of oxygen, nourishment, and liquids. He would call my mom with every update.

CHAPTER 6

Cautiously Optimistic

AT MY BEDSIDE, Dad started to read the book titled *The Law of Love* by Nora Roberts to me. The nurses told him that I was aware and could hear and that any stimulus would help my brain. While I was not moving much, barely had one eye open at times, and was not speaking, he still knew I was listening. Several months later he quizzed me on the book's title, its author, and the protagonist's name, which was also Sara, and I could recall them all. He told me later that there were some love scenes in the book, which he didn't feel very comfortable reading to me as my dad, so he tended to "gloss over" those sections. Dad said he felt really bad for me because I had big bandages at the front and back of my head and tubes everywhere—two down my throat and several attached to both arms. He could see how painful it was for me, whenever they moved me, which they needed to do every few hours to prevent any bed sores.

My mom returned on June 22. While she had been gone, the doctors performed a tracheotomy to help me breathe. I have a permanent scar on my neck now. They basically sliced a hole in my neck and put a breathing tube down my throat. Since I could not control my saliva and swallow functions, the medical staff was using the trach to suction the saliva out of my throat and prevent me from choking. The trach tube also gave me another airway to breathe. In addition to the trach, I was also put on a ventilating machine for a couple of weeks. At times they would ramp the ventilator up, so my breathing was comparable to what I would have during a light jog. My chest would move up and down quickly, as the oxygen was pumped into me. They told me they needed to do this to help decrease the pressure in my brain. It's hard for me to imagine my family seeing me pumped with air, while still lying unresponsive in a hospital bed.

A month after the stroke, when my body had stabilized, I graduated from the ICU and was moved into a recovery center. My mom constantly asked the doctor when my trach could be downsized or removed altogether, as she thought it was becoming unnecessary. As the weeks went by, I was more able to control my saliva and swallowing functions. To make matters worse, the nurses were very quick to "suction," as they call it, while I had the trach in, by using a little tube or vacuum type gadget to suck up excess saliva that I couldn't swallow. One time a nurse actually suctioned me too deeply and drew blood. After that, my mom would tell everyone who took care of me that I didn't need to be suctioned and I now had a very strong cough, and it would prevent me from choking. She even waited until the overnight staff arrived to tell them not to suction me. I'm grateful that my mom tried to protect me this way. I never understood it when other patients would motion to be suctioned because I hated it. It was painful and irritating. It would always make me cough, and my entire body would become tense, as the suction tube made my gag reflex contract. My face would turn red, and my body would become very tense. It was extremely irritating.

It was in the ICU where the staff determined I was well enough to discharge. Some physical therapists came in my room, pulled me into a sitting position and "dangled" me, by dangling my legs over a bed. Of course, I flopped like a rag doll. I had no muscle tone, no strength anywhere and no voluntary movement. My spine could not hold me up, and my neck muscles could not support my head. The doctors told my parents that I was not a candidate for rehab at that time.

One thing I do remember about the ICU is the big blue boots they put on my feet to prevent "foot drop." When you have to stay lying down too much, your feet can become deformed in the bed as the Achilles heel tightens. Foot drop would have frozen my feet in a position that would have prevented me from walking normally, so in hindsight I'm glad I wore the boots. Yet at the time, I hated them because they were so uncomfortable. My parents put them on me every night during my rehab, and my feet always really hurt the next morning. I don't know why because they didn't hurt when they first were put on, and as odd as it sounds I could actually sleep fine in them, but by morning, I was always in pain. Because I couldn't speak, I wasn't able to ask them to take the boots off in the morning and that was very frustrating. I was in pain; but I was not able to tell anyone how to help me.

Also during the early part of my ER stay, they surgically put a G-tube (feeding tube), in my stomach and fed me that way for a couple of months. I have a permanent scar on my stomach from it still today. I had a tube going into my neck, stomach, and bladder when my mom returned. You can imagine how unexcited she was about all that. She immediately made it her personal mission to "unhook" me and get me back home to Wisconsin.

At the end of June, I was moved into the Topanga Terrace Recovery Center, a month after my stroke, but the only thing that I could move on my body was my right pinky finger. When it moved ever so slightly, everyone became very excited. I guess that not being able to move anything and then moving my finger was a lot for everyone to witness.

I would like to give my personal recognition to all the care-givers in the world. They are all remarkable. Personally, I believe I had the best caregivers on the planet. I have never met anyone else who has acted as selflessly as my parents did during my stroke recovery.

They flew out to California from Wisconsin immediately upon receiving the doctor's call. No questions asked. They stayed with me through it all. I took them away from their lives for nearly six months! Their coming to California was only the beginning of their help. They continued to help me daily to recover in Wisconsin too. I am incredibly grateful to have such wonderful parents, and to have had these amazing caregivers throughout my rehab.

Because my parents were helping every day, I noticed other caregivers more often and respect them a lot as well. I also be-lieve my parents were actually kind of lucky as caregivers because they always had more concrete belief that I'd get better. Many caregivers don't have that same level of hope, but they are still very patient and loving every day. I admire them enormously. Remember, there is ALWAYS hope!

CHAPTER 7

Transition out of ICU

I WAS IN the Intensive Care Unit (ICU) for about twenty days. That is the highest level of life-saving care possible. The hospital then put me in a regular room on a different floor for a week in the same hospital. Then, the doctors said I needed to leave the hospital, in so many words, because they had saved my life and stabilized me. So my mom, Dad, Peter, and my friend Cary, started to look for another place where I could start the next phase of my recovery. My mom questioned why they would discharge a non-verbal paralyzed patient who required so much care, but the hospital was insistent that I needed to go somewhere else. My life was going to change again and I had no control of it. My parents, Cary and Peter visited eight facilities and chose Topanga Terrace because it was the "cleanest and brightest" and had the "youngest staff." I lived there for three months from June 2009 until September 2009.

They also kept a personal journal for me and my ongoing accomplishments. This became very special to me. They would write down what I did each day and date it. They detailed everything: my moving a leg, what I ate, any visitors, etc. I know it doesn't sound like much, but I still treasure this journal. I couldn't see my progress, so it was good for me to look at this journal and prove to myself how far I'd come. For example, I could say "Hey, on July 11, 2009 everyone was excited because I could pick up my right foot and put it down." Obviously, that's not a big deal, but at the time it was. One of my favorite entries is when my dad was making my stuffed bunny, Connie, do exercises for me. I can still picture this activity in my head, and I think it's really cute. My parents also kept a "guestbook" for visitors to write me messages. This was, of course, very special too.

My parents left everything to be with me. My dad is a retired teacher, and he gave up all his time to be with me. My mom was not yet retired and was still a rural mail carrier in LaCrosse, Wisconsin. She had saved up her sick days and vacation days from thirty years, so she could come and be with me. They both had their own lives, houses, and grandchildren who they left to be with me. For that, I will be eternally grateful.

Because of their sacrifices, I was relieved to be able to return to Wisconsin because I felt guilty about taking them away from their lives. However, whenever I mentioned anything about it to them, they always assured me that everything was okay. My dad would even say "I actually feel lucky to be with you because I hardly see you anymore!" I felt the same about seeing them. I knew it wasn't the situation any of us would have wanted or planned, but I wanted them to know that I was very sorry for everything, and I truly appreciated everything they did for me out of nothing but pure love.

Once we returned home to Wisconsin after six months in three different recovery centers, I was still 100 percent dependent on my parents. I was in a wheelchair, so they had to help me with everything! Cooking, cleaning, dressing, everything! I lived with my mom during this time, but my dad would come over daily and make me breakfast. Then I would practice my handwriting, and then Dad would help me walk. At first, I walked with a walker, then a cane, but eventually, I transitioned to a no-assistive device. Dad would walk behind me and hold the gait belt that was always around my waist during the day in case I got off balance, which I often did.

I can't imagine what it was like for my dad to come over to the house we had all once lived in together, and which he originally helped build. But still, he would come over most days a week to get me up and strengthen my atrophied body. This was necessary because my mom had gone back to work. Although she had saved up thirty years of sick days and vacation days to be with me in California, she still was not receiving her full salary, so financially she needed to go back to work.

Both of my parents were always there whenever I broke down emotionally, which I often did early on in my rehab. After the stroke, I would cry a lot. I would cry because the whole situation was sad and unfair, and I was very scared about what the future would hold for me. Everything in life was a big question mark. Anytime we saw a doctor about anything, the doctor's response was always "I don't know, so let's give it more time." I understood that they didn't want to be accountable, but I still thought *You're the doctor! You should tell me what to expect!*

It was very frustrating. Mom would remind me of her calm feelings to reassure me that everything would be okay. Dad didn't really know what to do when I would cry, but he would always remind me that I wasn't "stealing his time." That was something I often worried about.

They visited me in California from 9 a.m. to 7 p.m. every day. In Wisconsin, my parents also took me to therapy on Mondays, Wednesdays and Fridays at Gundersen Hospital or the University of Wisconsin-LaCrosse, in LaCrosse, Wisconsin, a forty-minute drive each way. There were other kinds of therapy later that they took me to as well. Examples of these are: hippotherapy (horse therapy), yoga, swimming, reflexology. Both were kind of like my "cheerleaders" during therapy. They would watch everything carefully and mentally take notes to record what I did.

I don't think I can ever do or say enough to truly thank my parents for all that they've done for me, but I am eternally grateful to them. They never left me. I know how much they had to sacrifice to be with me, and I know there is nothing I could possibly say or write to completely express my full gratitude to them. Apart from the innumerable characteristics about them that I admire, I also appreciated their honesty and sincerity with me. For example, they never gave me a compliment on my progress if I didn't deserve it, and I loved that truth. When they gave me a compliment, I really felt I had earned it. I had a hard time seeing my own progress, which can be so hard when you need to maintain your own motivation, so I blindly believed them. I also realize that no one wanted to trade places with them during this time, but they treated me just like you would want and hope parents would treat an adult child in my situation.

They are both my lifelong heroes. If I am ever fortunate

enough to become a parent, I hope I can be even half as great as my parents have been. I know I wouldn't have recovered nearly as well without them nearby and without their love, encouragement and support. Hopefully this chapter in my book thanks them in some small formal way.

CHAPTER 8

More Angels

VEN THOUGH I was unconscious, I know I had the best visitors in the world when I was sick and while I was recovering. As you may have noticed, I've started these last chapters similarly, but my statements are totally sincere. I am very blessed to have amazing people around me. Even Dad once told me, "You have more friends than anyone I've known in my entire life!" I thought that was pretty cool of him to say. My friends were all shocked to hear the news of my stroke. They weren't just worried about me; they were also worried about my parents. I will try here to describe my friends and visitors as best I can.

First of all, my boyfriend at the time, Peter, knew he had to alert our closest friends to my critical condition. He did so by sending the following email.

> Friends—With sad news, my girlfriend of two years, Sara Anderson, suffered a major stroke last Wednesday, June 3rd. She has been in the intensive care unit ever since. She had three brain procedures in seventy-two hours and is hanging on to life. The situation is very serious and highly concerning. She is twenty-seven years old and the most health-conscious individual I know. Sara has been unconscious for the past six days, but today she showed signs of hope with some movements. Despite also fighting a fever and a lung infection, the medical staff feels Sara's vital signs have mostly been stabilized and that she will survive. While Sara is not "awake," doctors believe she is partially conscious, can hear us, and is making slight efforts to open her eyes. She has responded to some simple commands, such as "squeeze my right hand" and "wiggle your toes." She is still on a breathing ventilator. The doctors say probably it will be another seven to ten days (or longer) before the swelling goes down in her brain, and she begins to wake up. Not until then can her condition be truly determined. She needs time, and of course lots of love and support. It's a long road ahead. For Sara, I ask for your prayers and good energy. Love Peter

My very first friends to come and visit me at the hospital were Debbi and Lauren, two of my best friends from school in Wisconsin. They bought a plane ticket immediately when they heard the news and arrived the next day for an overnight visit. Debbi was still even nursing her daughter, Tammi! Tammi joined her and thus took her first plane trip. On their flight, they were praying that I would stay alive. They were both disappointed that it took a medical emergency for them to visit me in LA for the first time. It was not the visit that we had always imagined.

When they arrived at the hospital, they gave all my family big hugs, as they were familiar with each other. They also greatly sympathized with my parents, who were so concerned for my well-being in the Intensive Care Unit, and they were happy to see that everyone around me loved me so much. "Can we see and talk to Sara?" They asked.

"Yes, she's right in here. But she's unable to respond."

"That's okay."

They then entered my ICU room. Mom tried to prepare them about my condition. Obviously, I looked a lot different than the last time they had seen me only a few weeks earlier during my visit at home in Wisconsin. Seeing me comatose and unresponsive and connected to so many machines was hard for everyone. They desperately wanted their friend back. They returned to Wisconsin the next day and they continued saying prayers for me all the way.

Debbi deserves special recognition for being such a good friend to me. Unfortunately, we had fallen a bit out of touch since high school while she was busy getting married and creating beautiful children and I was busy traveling the world. However, when this tragedy struck me, despite my being out of touch with her, she was there for me in a heartbeat. Later, when I was back in Wisconsin, she really made an effort to be there for me. She invited me to multiple social gatherings and even for weekends away at her timeshare. While we attended school together in Westby (population 2,200), Debbi is from an even smaller local town called Chaseburg (population 296), about 15 to 20 minutes away by car. However, I regularly saw Debbi after the stroke, mostly from her visits to my house in Westby. When we were in school, Debbi and I were "partners in crime" and we can be very goofy when we are together. She didn't care about my stroke at all when it came to our friendship and she went out of her way to show me how much our friendship means to her. She is the truest friend that I've ever had.

My next visitors in the hospital were Lucienne and Reka, two fellow teachers and friends of mine from USC. Together they visited me in the ICU. Being mothers themselves, they greatly empathized with my parents and their scary situation. My parents bonded with both women and enjoyed their company, and they visited me regularly at the recovery center. They helped my mom get in contact with my boss at USC who could help in this emergency situation. He gave my mom a list of contacts to help figure out what to do for me. Everyone at USC was amazing to my family and me during this tragic situation. I really appreciated that they kept my friends at USC up to date on what was happening to me as time progressed.

The next to visit me was my friend Terry. I originally met Terry while I was in Hawaii earning my Master's degree, as he was also. Terry is originally from Shanghai, China. He moved to New York City when I moved to Los Angeles. Then, one year later, he moved to LA. I was happy to have him in LA to hang out with again. I helped him look for an apartment when he first moved to town. Terry came to the ICU to visit me a couple of times, and it was very emotional for him. He was thoughtful and brought authentic Chinese food from LA's Chinatown for my parents, and they ate together in the waiting room. I feel incredibly grateful to have Terry in my life.

Next, my friend Cary visited me from Hawaii. Like Terry, I originally met Cary while I was in Hawaii earning my Master's degree, as was she. Cary has a son, Kai, and the three of us would often go to the beach or go for a jog or just hang out. Cary immediately bought a plane ticket after she heard about my stroke. She was very upset about my condition, particularly as I was not responding much nor speaking during her first visit to see me.

On her first day of visiting, Cary said, "Kai is very upset with me because he knows I'm visiting Auntie Sara, but I didn't bring him." Kai had sent a little turtle or "honu," as it's called in the Hawaiian language. He remembered that I loved turtles when I lived in Hawaii. The little stuffed turtle became a permanent fixture in my hospital bed. Kai also sent a get-well card with a voice recording inside it that said "Hi Sara, it's Kai. Hope you feel better soon! You rock!" It was really sweet. I still remember listening to it. Cary and Kai both visited me in California in November 2009, right when I was being discharged from the hospital. It was great to see them both again. At that time, I was still in a wheelchair. Cary helped me do floor exercises, and we had great fun catching up, as now I could talk quietly. Cary is definitely one of my best friends and since she still lives in Honolulu, I told her that I intend to wear out my welcome visiting her, particularly during the months of January and February, when winter is at its worst in Wisconsin.

Another of my closest friends from the University of Hawaii who visited me was Rachel. Terry, Cary, Rachel and I were all good friends in Hawaii. We met each other while earning our master's degrees in the same Second Language Studies program at the University. Rachel and I especially bonded when we were selected to teach an Intensive Summer English program at the Kyoto Women's University in Kyoto, Japan. We were roommates in Japan and again "partners in crime." I'll leave the stories out, but they could probably be a great book all by themselves! Whenever I think of Rachel, I always smile because we have a similar sense of humor. She always makes me laugh, and we have our own inside jokes that only the two of us understand. She knows Portuguese and Spanish and instead of teaching ESL, she is a Spanish and Portuguese teacher now at the University of Hawaii at Mānoa. Rachel visited me twice during my recovery in California. On her first visit, I was still in the ICU. She was just returning to the U.S., after teaching in Venezuela for a while that summer. Her second visit was in September of 2009 when I was in the Topanga nursing home. I could interact a bit more the second time. She always brought a smile to my face and a laugh out of me. Rachel and I have many inside jokes, and I am still so happy the stroke didn't affect my memory of our stories.

I know some of my friends would be disappointed if I didn't describe "the knot" that was in my hair. (Many people tried to gently brush it out, but with little success.) Before my mom went back to Wisconsin for her radiation treatment, she tried to brush out as much of my hair as she could. Then she braided it, so it wouldn't get tangled while she was gone. However, the remaining hair on the other side of my incision (which she could not reach because of the attached machines) was where "the knot" formed. There was a nurse named Connie in the ICU and she kind of took me under her wing. She also noticed my long hair and "the knot" and told her daughter about me. Her little girl asked, "Mommy is she like Rapunzel?" "Yes, she is," Connie replied.

Nurse Connie even used her own money to buy me a brush, conditioner and de-tangler to try to soak and loosen the knot in my hair. It didn't work, and "the knot" just got tighter, but it was very thoughtful of her. My parents were truly touched by her kindness, and I was too when they told me about it. Another friend, Natalie, was brushing my hair once and she knew I was in pain. She said, "Sara, they want to shave your head like Sinead O'Connor, and right now you kind of look like Bob Marley, so squeeze my hand if you want me to continue to brush your hair."

I hadn't responded much in the ICU up to that point, but Natalie says she definitely felt me squeeze her hand, so she kept brushing, as I had "instructed." "The knot" was so tight that when my mom returned, she couldn't even put the tip of her manicure scissors in it. We never got it all brushed out despite all the effort my friends made. So my mom simply pulled down my hair as far as she could and cut out that knot–strand by strand. The rest of my hair disguised it so you couldn't even see it, as it was growing out.

My most impressive visitor was my Grandma Anderson, because she had never been on a plane in her entire life. Then she did it twice to come see me. When she was talking to my dad one night over the phone, she told him, "Gary, it looks like I'll be getting on an airplane after all." She was accompanied by my Uncle Keith and my aunts Tricia, Ann, and Marilyn. They felt really bad for my parents and me, but they were also very encouraging at the same time. When I returned to Wisconsin, they would drive from Iowa to visit me about once a month, and again they were always so encouraging when they saw me. I remember on one of these visits that I complimented Grandma Anderson on doing such a good job raising Dad. I said the same thing to my Grandma Sieber about Mom. I was in awe of these very strong characters in my life. My Dad's family all live in Carpenter, Iowa. It is a very small town with a population of 1073, even smaller than Westby where I grew up. It is also about three hours away from Westby. Grandma would often make me delicious baked goods until I went on a diet and asked her to stop. She means so much to me, and her wonderful support was greatly appreciated.

A couple of months prior to my stroke, my brother Brian and my sister-in-law Melanie were the only family members who had visited me in LA before the stroke. After the stroke, they came to California twice to see me. The first time, they came right away with my parents when I was in the ICU. They came a second time when I was in the nursing home during an emotional low I was having. I was very confused that the stroke and its aftermath that were truly happening to me. I was trapped in a hospital bed with little movement and little speech.

On August 24 my mom had told me that my Grandpa Sieber had passed away, and she had to leave for a week to go to his funeral. I loved him so much, but I couldn't be at his funeral, and that was very hard for me to accept. In fact, I couldn't believe that he had died. My mom wanted Brian and Melanie, who were in California with me, to stay with me during this time instead of returning for the funeral. It was very nice and reassuring to have them by my side, encouraging me and helping me come to terms with the stroke. It was hard while my mother was gone. I kept thinking I was only in a nightmare, and I kept asking Brian, Melanie and everyone around me how to wake up from that nightmare. When my mother returned after my Grandpa's funeral, I realized for the first time that my situation was real and maybe I was not dreaming at all.

My sister Lisa, and my nephews, Tyler and Tanner, and my niece, Isabella, also came to see me in the ICU along with my parents. Lisa and her kids had plans to come back in August, but that didn't work out unfortunately because my Grandpa died the day before their flight. I had a wonderful surprise when my cousin, Jamie, visited. I hadn't seen Jamie in years. Growing up, I only saw my cousins, Ricky and Jamie, my Aunt Sue's children, every few years because of the distance between our home in Wisconsin and theirs in Texas. Jamie was on a summer road trip with his cousins, and while driving through LA, he came to visit me in the nursing home. He was studying to become a doctor. He looked so good! He had lost a lot of weight since the last time I had seen him. I was unable to speak at the time of his visit, but he talked to Mom and Dad, so I listened to his conversation with my parents. I appreciated his visit very much.

I was surprised later when I realized that so many of my family and friends knew each other. My memory is almost non-existent about my hospital ICU stay. I don't even remember my family. Later, when I would talk about people, I would discover that certain people already knew each other. This was odd for me because I had no memory of their ever meeting. While I thought it was strange, I was still happy that the closest people in my life actually knew each other.

My doctors knew I would have a tough time emotionally coming to grips with the stroke, so after a few months, they arranged for a miracle stroke rehabber to visit me. That beautiful miracle was Jen. Although I was just meeting her for the first time, I was very grateful to have her as part of my recovery. Jen had also suffered a stroke from the same combination of birth control pills with migraines and aura, and she was an amazing resource for me. I know that all strokes are different, but ours were very similar in several ways. We were both twenty-seven at the age of our strokes and suffered from migraines with aura; we were also on combined estrogen and progesterone birth control pills.

One big difference between our strokes is that Jen's was diagnosed faster (because she passed out on her bathroom floor and her boyfriend called 911). She was immediately administered the tPA (tissue plasminogen activator) shot, the "clotbusting drug," upon reaching the ER, so she avoided having to have cranial surgery. My stroke, however, was slowing killing me while I sat in the waiting room of the ER for nearly five hours. Then, when the doctors quickly knocked me unconscious with morphine, it became impossible to diagnose the stroke, so my brain was stroking and dying for over fourteen hours before I received any help. The tPA shot could have saved much of my brain. I often wonder what my reality would have been had I not been forced to wait so long in the waiting room, or if I had been properly diagnosed and administered the shot like Jen. Amazingly enough, only three to four percent of all stroke victims are ever given this tPA shot. I must again restate that progesterone-only birth control is the "safest" form of birth control and that you should absolutely call 911 in an emergency in hopes of receiving the clot-busting drug in time.

Our neurologists actually worked together in the ICU, and Jen, after recovering, told her neurologist that she was willing to meet other stroke sufferers to help encourage them. She was referred to me, and we have been friends ever since. She is really remarkable. Jen had her stroke two years before I did, but you would never know she had even had one, even though she had to fight to get her motor skills and particularly her speech back. Because of this struggle, she was a true beacon of hope to my parents and, of course, also to me. I remembered seeing her in the nursing home when she was nearly two years into recovery. Later when I was two years recovered from my stroke, I was much farther away from my goals in my rehab goals, which was very depressing. I had to remind myself that Jen received the tPA shot, but I didn't. I believe that was a huge difference. I again realized the importance of the TIME IS BRAIN warnings for stroke treatment that you often see.

I remember once when Jen visited, she said that when people said the word "soon" to her, the meaning was ambiguous. That was exactly how I felt. I realized that everyone has a different interpretation of the word "soon." People would often say "Sara, you'll get better soon." I didn't know what that meant. I thought tomorrow would be good, but did "soon" mean next week? Next month? Next year? "Soon" held a great deal of subjectivity. When I was finishing my recovery in Wisconsin, I would keep in touch with Jen to maintain contact with her and ask her stroke-related questions. I put Jen on a high pedestal and hoped I could one day be recovered like she was. With that said, I still didn't feel ready to meet other stroke sufferers and share my own story until much later in my recovery. In honesty, I thought I may frighten them instead of inspire them as Jen had done for me, since I had so much further to go in my own recovery. However, I do give credit to Jen as she was the first person who inspired me to work so hard.

Many therapy dogs visited me during my time in the recovery centers. At Topanga, my most frequent visitor was Maddie, a miniature schnauzer, who visited Topanga every week. Maddie is an official "therapy dog" and had her own little red vest, which read "therapy dog." Maddie was very spoiled and was usually pushed around in a baby stroller. Mom said her paws rarely touched the ground. Maddie's owner was proud that Maddie had been featured on calendars. I really enjoyed Maddie's visits. At Northridge Hospital, I signed up again for visits from therapy dogs. Laddie and Wizard then visited me once a week. Laddie is a beautiful golden retriever. Wizard is a Portuguese water dog and supposedly a hypoallergenic dog breed. Overall, I always enjoyed the visits from these therapy dogs as it took my mind off my slow recovery. Of course, I was very much physically limited during their visits, thus limiting our interactions. However, the therapy dogs' helpers understood this.

My face would always light up into a big smile when they would greet me at the door, and then the helpers would lead the dog over to my bed so I could pet the dog's head with my right hand. Sometimes the dogs seemed extra interested in my left (more affected) side. I thought it was interesting to see how they could see how that was wounded on my body. The dogs were always very laid back and gentle. The visits of the therapy dogs were always very brief, of course, but I always really looked forward to seeing the dogs. They definitely lifted my spirits, which was the intention. If you have a loved one in the hospital who is also an animal lover, see if there are therapy dog visits.

As soon as I could speak, I asked my parents to please stop allowing human visitors to come to the recovery center. I did this because I was now becoming more conscious of my condition and my appearance, and I was now very embarrassed and insecure. I knew how people remembered me, and I was far away from what I was then. I was not comfortable with people seeing me in a lesser state of being. With that said, I limited my visits at the recovery center to my family during the last couple of months of my recovery in Los Angeles.

When I returned to Wisconsin, I had spent six months living in three different LA medical facilities. I didn't want to see anyone, as I was embarrassed and insecure. Still, I give my hometown friends a lot of credit for giving me the space I wanted and needed after my return to Westby. I didn't feel any pressure from them to have a visit, which I appreciated. I know it was hard for them not to come and see me. Some of my friends even admitted to doing "drive bys" of my mom's house, where I was living, to send good thoughts mentally to me for my quick recovery.

A number of months later, I eventually did contact four of my nearby friends, as I was ready; I found it was really nice to see everyone again. I saw Debbi and Lauren, who had visited me in the hospital in LA, and Tanya and Kelly, two more of my high school friends. At our initial reunion, the girls and I had a good reunion and then a good visit catching up on what had happened in the last six months. The ice was broken now, and it was much easier for me to keep in touch and see them from time to time. Even though I was still insecure about how I looked and how they remembered me, I learned that they were just happy I was still alive and loved me unconditionally as my friends.

Father Cook also visited me once I arrived home. Father Cook was the priest at our church in the nearby town of Viroqua. He helped my mother enormously after my stroke. I thought it was truly kind that he stopped over to see me, talk to me, and extend his best wishes, prayers and support to encourage me during my recovery.

I really tried my best to stay positive throughout my recovery, but honestly, I think now that my stroke could have been prevented if the doctors had not prescribed a combined estrogen and progesterone birth control since I was a migraine-with-aura sufferer, and this combination of medication is contra-indicated. I really hope that other people will avoid the same catastrophe that I experienced by being better informed about this terrible combination. Knowing that my story can help others has made my journey towards recovery even more worthwhile. I almost died due to my medication, and my doctors and pharmacist should have caught this error in advance and alerted me to it. So let my awful experience be a lasting example of how much you do have to be your own advocate for your own healthcare.

I am sure that it is obvious how grateful I am to have had such a wonderful support system from my family and friends that I have remembered in this chapter and many more. I am so proud of everyone for embracing me as much as they did and for being brave and patient with me. I know I was embarrassed, ashamed and insecure in my recovery, but when I was finally ready to face the world again, I also knew that I had many people cheering loudly and nonstop for me. I am overwhelmed by the amount of love that still surrounds me.

CHAPTER 9

Caringbridge.org

HILE DISCUSSING MY support system, I must describe how great my Caringbridge.org website was during my recovery. This website hosts profiles for people with health issues and updates are posted by the family detailing their progress. Family and friends are able to join the website and receive an email alert whenever an update is posted. There is also a guestbook for people, so they can leave a note for the person with the health issue.

I had heard about this website often from my parents' conversations each other about it after my stroke, but I didn't know what it was. When I returned to Wisconsin, I decided to see what "Sara's Caringbridge website" was all about, so I sat in a chair with my laptop and began to read. It took me at least two days to read it all! I was blown away by the updates and the guestbook submissions to say the least. Mom set a box of Kleenex next to me whenever she knew I was reading it. Remember, I grew up in a very small town where it seems like everyone knows everyone. It seemed now like the whole town was keeping up with me! I heard from people in my guestbook that I hadn't heard from since high school! It was really remarkable to read their support for me.

My sister in-law, Melanie, started the webpage because she didn't want my family to be overwhelmed with phone calls. She had been introduced to Caringbridge.org earlier, and she started the site hoping someone would take it over. Peter, my boyfriend at the time, ended up taking it over since he had more of the details and better access to information. He was with me almost every day when I stayed at the LA hospitals. He would write journal entries to keep everyone informed on my recovery, and people would leave me little notes of encouragement in the guestbook to let me know they were rooting for me. Everyone appreciated the updates. They wanted to stay informed even though many were geographically at a distance from me. I included some of the journal entries, but I left out the guestbook because it's difficult to choose them; they're all very special to me.

Top of Form Tuesday, June 9, 2009 10:39 AM, CDT (my stroke happened on June 3, 2009) Journal entry by Melanie Anderson — Jun 9, 2009:

"I am Sara's sister-in-law, Melanie. You will probably receive updates from several people. I'll begin where this all started from my stand point, and we will go from there. I was saying good-bye to my husband and Sara's brother, Brian, on Thursday morning,

June 4, when the call came at 6:40 a.m. As he took it, I could hear his mother, frantic on the other end, telling him that Sara had had a stroke. What happened after that is a blur, but we threw some bags together and 8 of us headed up to the twin cities to catch the 12:30 flight to L.A.

I remember very little of when we arrived, but I will get to what you want to hear. Peter will probably be able to give you more details, but I will tell you what I know. Sara and Peter had been at a hospital for several hours because Sara had had a migraine that she described as different from ones she usually experienced. After much waiting she was given some morphine and drifted off to sleep. The problem came when it was time to wake up. She didn't. The doctors gave her more time. Still, she didn't wake up. After a ct scan one doctor saw no irregularities, then two doctors, finally a third doctor at Kaiser Permanente saw something and said to get her there as soon as possible.

It was a stroke on the right side of her cerebellum, where her most basic of functions begin, in particular her internal alarm clock. At that point she was moving very little. We, her mom, dad, sister, brother, sis-in-law, 2 nephews and her niece, arrived and began talking to her, all of us along with her boyfriend Peter and his mom, dad, and brother, and encouraging her to move and wake up. And she did move. She let us know she was there and she could hear us. We were given hope.

The next few days were critical and very, very difficult and nerve-racking. On Friday she had two surgeries. The first was in the morning. Surgeons removed a piece of bone in the back of her skull to make room for the brain to swell. When she successfully made it through that procedure we were overjoyed. Our spirits began to rise until a phone call at dinner came to tell us she needed another surgery, a tiny hole drilled in her head where a catheter was place to drain some of the fluid that was building on her brain. This too was successful, and after a very hard day we all slept a little more peacefully knowing that she was now getting a little better.

On Saturday she rested with very little change as I remember and in the words of the doctor, we were still not out of the woods.

On Sunday, Sara had developed a slight fever, which the doctors were controlling and they had found a spot on the lung-pneumonia or an infection of some sort developed from having her respirator in. But still, on that day we heard the words, cautiously optimistic. These were the first positive things the doctors had to say.

On Monday, while she still had a fever and the infection, the doctors definitely seemed less grim when they spoke to us. They began using words like 'recovery.' Before when we had asked they said not to talk about it. We really felt by this time, Sara had turned a corner. At this point she is responding to simple commands such as 'squeeze my right hand' and 'wiggle your toes.' She's moving her extremities for us and blinking her eyes and even at times opening one eye.

What is happening to her as the doctors tell us (and this will be hard for you to hear) is that she's trapped inside her body. She is conscious, aware, and can hear us. She knows that we are there. Her road will be long. The doctors say probably seven to ten days before the swelling goes down in her brain and she begins to wake up. And perhaps longer. But it will happen. Injuries of the brain take longer to heal than other injuries. She just needs time. And lots of love and support of course.

On a side note, you will notice on the right side of the page a place to make a donation. Please note that this donation does not go to the Anderson family, but to the caringbridge website to give to who they want. If you wish to do something for Sara and her family, please contact me.

My email address is ladyflutterby@hotmail.com.

And finally, thank you for your prayers. Each and every one is helping her. Continue to pray for her recovery.

Thank you!"

Much of this caring bridge web copy was emotionally difficult to read, but especially the early days, reading about what my family went through was especially difficult. I know the doctor said I was aware, but I have no memory of these early days. Therefore, it was difficult to relive them through my family's eyes.

Tuesday, June 23, 2009 8:05 PM, CDT "Journal entry by Melanie Anderson — Jun 23, 2009 Hello everyone!

Great news! The results from Sara's MRI are back. The thinking part of her brain is undamaged and they said her prognosis for recovery looks very good. I don't have much more to tell you at the moment, but I thought you would want to know. Our prayers are working:) Melanie."

I think this is significant because it describes how my thinking was undamaged. While I had to recover a lot still, I was always so grateful not to have lost my cognition (which would have included the loss of all of my education), my memory, and my language.

Sunday, August 30, 2009 8:47 PM, CDT By: Peter Sara Update 8/30

"Friends of Sara —

With great respect, I would first like to recognize Mr. Robert Sieber, Sara's Grandfather, who sadly passed away this last Monday, August 24. The loss has been a most difficult one for the

Sieber / Anderson family. I know all of our hearts and good wishes go out to the family.

Last year, I had the privilege to meet Mr. Sieber at his home in LaCrosse. We talked about life and football and I got to hear an interesting war story or two. A real gentleman and storyteller he was. I also know how much he meant to Sara. Mr Sieber will be fondly remembered by all that admired him so dearly. We are now at three months since Sara's incident. Sara has continued to make some important improvements over the past two weeks. Step by step she climbs the difficult mountain toward recovery. Many miles to go, but her forward momentum continues.

Big news—Sara had her trach tube removed from her throat. She now has full control of her breathing and swallowing. The transition has been very smooth.

With the trach removed, Sara is now whispering words and short sentences. The whispering started as very faint sounds and has now evolved into communication. While still very quiet, her volume seems to be increasing with time. She is whispering quite a bit and our communication with her has vastly improved. She whispers quickly and not everything is audible, but it certainly is getting better as she gets more control of speaking. We do hear her actual voice at times, but for the most part it is whispers. We feel she is on the verge of regaining a louder voice soon, which will make a big difference for her psyche and our continued communication.

Sara has a good appetite and is being spoon-fed three times a day, plus she is getting some food-fiber from her feeding tube. Her menu will soon expand to more soft foods, as she is improving with chewing and swallowing. Some food variance will certainly make her happier.

Sara is attempting to help feed herself by working on fork and spoon movements, as well as with drinking cup movements. In short time, the therapists will help her fine tune her coordination with feeding/drinking utensils.

Sara's neck soreness seems to be gone. She is now rotating her neck side to side. She still needs more neck strength to fully control her neck motions and to hold her head up and steady when being sat and stood up, but it's coming with time.

Sara's shoulders also seem to be on the mend. She is now doing exercises to roll her shoulders. The right shoulder has recovered quicker and is no longer taped. The left remains taped, but seems on its way to recovery.

Sara continues to do daily therapy and is building more consistency and strength.

We have been most impressed that her left side is starting to wake up a bit more. As mentioned previously, her left side seems to be quite behind her right side in recovery. However, like her right leg, her left leg is now doing slow leg lifts and retractions, which is fantastic to see. Her left fingers and hand are starting to slowly move a bit more. Her left arm has not moved much, but it's something the therapists will now focus on to spark a return.

Also to our amazement, Sara has had 1.5 lb. weights put on both ankles as she does some lower leg kicks (knee to foot), while sitting at the side of the bed. This exercise, to swing the leg, is important to build strength in consideration of the walking process.

Building more trunk strength is a main goal right now, so Sara can stand with more balance and comfort.

Big News: Each day this week, Sara has been stood up with a tall walker in front of her. With the assistance of two to three therapists, she has started to take tiny steps across the floor. She can manage six to ten small steps per session with assistance (one person helping to hold and balance her body, one person to help guide her kick / feet, one person to watch her head / neck). With each time, Sara gains a bit more comfort and confidence. She still needs more trunk control, balance and coordination, but it's certainly a start! At first it was scary for her, but now she has a look of determination and amazement as she attempts tiny steps. It brings tears of hope to us each day.

Sara's right eye remains half to three-quarters open. She will see an eye-doctor in mid September. We hope her visual issues will largely be corrected in time, as the eye nerves and muscles regenerate and heal.

The last few weeks have continued to be very emotional for Sara, as she becomes more in tune with her body and mind. Her emotions are certainly understandable under the circum- stances. Unfortunately her recovery is not a quick fix, but will take time and hard work. Now that she can communicate with words, her emotions are even more prevalent. We are doing all that we can to bring her calmness, understanding and focus.

We expect to hear soon about returning Sara to the hospital in early September for her ninety-day evaluation.

It's been very nice to have Sara's brother, Brian, and his wife, Melanie, here over the past week. Their visit has certainly been a great boost for Sara. Thanks for your continued good thoughts and prayers. I know you keep Sara in mind all the time, and for that we feel blessed and thankful. Peter"

This post is significant because it announces my Grandpa Sieber's death, which was also the start of when I began to think I was in a nightmare, truly the most terrifying period of my recovery. It also points out that I had begun "walking," even though I was using a walker with a therapist placing my feet. I didn't think this was impressive at the time, but reading back on it later, I can identify it as progress. It also notes that my tracheotomy tube was removed. I remember everyone being so excited that it was gone.

CHAPTER 10

Caringbridge.org (part II)

ARINGBRIDGE PLAYED SUCH a large and special role in my recovery, so appropriately, that story continues here. As in the previous chapter, I have offered some interesting journal entries that describe my therapy and my progress.

Monday, December 14, 2009 1:36 PM, CST

"Hello everyone, this is Sara. The purpose of this 'update' is to express all my gratitude to all of you who wrote me, checked up on me and prayed for me during this past six months. Many people have commented in the Guestbook, and I agree, that you never know how much life means until circumstances like this occur. And in this case, I am so fortunate to be alive to further know, and I hope all of you know too.

I am, of course, so grateful to have Peter in my life and to have had him provide all of the updates to those closest to me. And I know that I have such a great family to help me through this ordeal.

I would like to share a few details of what happened. Years ago I went on the birth control pill due to irregular periods. A few years later, I began to have migraine headaches with aura. I would always describe the aura as looking into a bright light then looking away, which would last about a ½ an hour before a headache ensued. My neurologist, who took care of me after the stroke, said my being female and having migraines combined with aura should have cautioned a doctor from prescribing me the Pill. Everyone takes the Pill so I didn't think anything dangerous about it. Mine was called Yasmin, supposedly a lower hormone alternative. I was also on medication called Midrin for migraines.

I typically got one migraine each month, but the week leading up to the stroke, I got a migraine every other day. What I did not know at the time, nor was alerted to, was that people taking both migraine meds and birth control are at higher risk for stroke. The combination when birth control thickens your blood can be dangerous and even deadly. The medications were prescribed to me by different doctors and refilled at the same time by the same pharmacist. Kaiser Hospital has electronic records and both doctors and the pharmacist failed to make the connection that the medicines carried contradictory warnings.

The week I had so many migraines I ran out of Midrin. My migraines were out of control so I called to make an appointment to see a migraine specialist, but I was told I needed a referral first, so it would take a few days. In the meantime, I ordered more migraine meds and on the same call I also ordered more Yasmin. They both were delivered to me a few days later, on the morning of my stroke.

Mostly my migraines were triggered by bright lights. On the day of the stroke, I first went to the gym. When I got home I went to take a shower, but I felt too light-headed to continue. I thought it may have been because of the bright ceiling lights at the gym. So I got out of the shower to try to regroup, but I felt weird. Thankfully, Peter was working from home that day. For those of you who don't know, Peter had just bought a house in LA and we had just moved in together. When I say just moved in, I mean just that: the stroke happened 6/3, we moved into the house 4/25, but were out of CA 5/10-5/20. I told him that it felt different and that my tongue felt numb. So we rushed immediately to 'urgent care' Kaiser (emergency ward) where we waited for hours to even be seen as it was so crowded. Peter helped do all he could to speed things along. We were finally admitted into an emergency doctor's room and hours later when the hospital figured out this was much more than a severe migraine, I was rushed into an emergency surgery. I then had two blood clots surgically removed from the back of my brain stem, which were blocking oxygen to my brain and thereby caused the stroke.

I was only twenty-seven, vegetarian, and very healthy. I worked out for an hour on the elliptical machine for a minimum three days a week and hiked with Peter on weekends. Now I'm confined to a wheelchair and have very limited use of my left hand. The scariest part for me was feeling like I was trapped in a bad dream. I really thought I was dreaming and couldn't wake up because I could not move nor speak. But it felt so real, too real. I even tried to act out of character to try to end the dream, but nothing worked. I didn't understand it or how this could be happening. A long time has passed and I absolutely appreciate all the good energy, support and prayers. I will need more while finishing my long recovery ahead. It is very hard for me to type (doing so with just my right pointer finger) so I am not answering email yet. Thank you doesn't even begin to express my gratitude to all of you. This really is the season to say I love you and I really do love all of you. Thank you an enormous amount!

Love to all—Sara"

I wrote this update shortly after my return to Wisconsin. I had just read Caringbridge for the first time, and I was astounded by the amount of support I saw I had received, after reading all of the journals and entries in the guestbook. I wanted to express the great amount of gratitude I felt and also alert everyone to the medications I was on which were the cause of my stroke. I didn't want anyone else to be using those two medications simultaneously. I later learned that the bigger concern was being a migraine sufferer with aura and taking a combined estrogen and progesterone birth control pill. I typed the message with one hand, but I was proud that I didn't have to dictate it to my parents for them to type.

Wednesday, December 29, 2010 10:28 AM, CST

By Sara Anderson 12/29/10

"Happy New Year! (I included a similar letter in my Christmas cards to my family this year.)

This is Sara. I wanted to send out an update since so many of you have kept up with me and for that I want to say THANK YOU! I truly appreciate all your love and prayers!

Well, it has been quite a year for me! It's about a year and a half since my stroke incident on June 3, 2009. After living in Los Angeles hospitals for six months, I arrived in Wisconsin from California on November 24, 2009. Let me review some of 2010 for you. I never would have guessed that I'd be living in Wisconsin again and certainly not under these circumstances, but I really enjoy being close to family and Wisconsin friends again. That is definitely the best part about being home; I receive endless amounts of love, support, and help from those around me. My parents are remarkable, and their courage and strength amaze me every day. They actually have turned into therapists to help me recover. Peter is also amazing. He has been able to visit every couple of months, and he is another wonderful source of love and support.

I want to talk about some of my achievements this past year, but I will preface it by saying that unfortunately, I am unable to see my progress. Maybe it is a matter of being too hard on myself, or that I am too close to everything, or that stroke recovery is so incredibly slow, but I often have to be told by others who don't see me every day how much I've improved. I honestly don't think I could possibly be working harder. I am doing therapy all day long, every day.

I am now practicing walking by myself, but it is very slow and deliberate. I began by using a walker, then I moved to a quad (four-point) cane, then a single-point cane, and then nothing. Initially, it was very scary to walk without any support. Imagine walking on a tightrope. That sensation of losing your balance and falling is similar to what I feel daily, but that fear is much less intense than it used to be. During the summer, my Dad and I began to walk around the high school track. At first it took me fifty-seven minutes for one lap, but now my best time was seventeen minutes. Nothing to brag about, but definitely, it is a big improvement for me.

I also had two eye surgeries in 2010 to help the alignment of my eyes. The stroke greatly affected my eye muscles, leaving my right eye stuck in the outer corner of my eye. I had no control over this situation, but it made it hard to see. Many therapists also thought it contributed to my body imbalance, and obviously the misalignment was very embarrassing for me physically. Both surgeries were very successful, however, and my eye alignment has been greatly improved. The success of these surgeries was a big highlight of 2010 for me.

When I began my therapy in Wisconsin, I was lacking some strength on my left side. However, on my last therapy check, my strength tested as normal. My brain just has to recognize that it is okay to use my left side again all the time.

My scheduled therapy at the hospital has stopped unfortunately, because the insurance stopped paying. I was going three days each week, but now I only go once every two months for a recheck. However, like I said, I am doing therapy all day every day, and despite not attending any scheduled therapy, I definitely feel like I'm getting my workout every day.

I love this time of the year because gratitude is so greatly emphasized. I feel that if I ad to sum up my emotions of 2010, I could do so with the one word 'gratitude.' I am so grateful for all that I have. Maybe that sounds odd, because of all I am still lacking, but that is my outlook. It is very depressing to think of what I could or should be doing, so I just try to focus on what I can do. I hope and pray that I can get back to where I was. I am stronger now than I was last year, and I know I have a long way to go, but I still have a strong personal motivation to work hard. I am very grateful for Caring Bridge as well. Thank you for all of your messages and encouragement. I read them all, and it is so nice to hear from all of you! It has now been about a year since I first read Caring Bridge. I was so surprised then, and I still am now just how many people are behind me. Thank you again for that! It is so nice to know you're all there for me.

There has been an incredible amount of therapy for me to do, and that will continue to be my future. We are hoping that hard work, time, prayers, and love will eventually bring me back to 'normal.' That is my ultimate goal. I would love nothing more than to pick up where I left off. Thank you for being a part of my life and for keeping up with my long journey back to being 'me'. Your love means the world to me! Love, Sara"

For this post, I wanted to provide a summary of some of my achievements for the previous year. I was so appreciative of my Caring Bridge support that I wanted to address everyone again. I left the updates to Peter because it was so difficult for me to type, and I struggled to see my progress. However, my mother decided to start "pre-approving" his journals when she felt they were not being as positive and supportive as they should be.

At this point in my recovery, I also went through a break-up when my boyfriend left me, so all entries after this one will be written by me.

Written May 15, 2013 7:24pm

"Hello all. This is Sara. Many of you already know this since I posted something similar on facebook, but I wanted you all to be aware since Peter was such an important part of caringbridge. Peter has ended our relationship. You may be as shocked as I was/am. This is a private matter. I will not offer any details here. If you want more details, please contact us directly. However, since I only type with 1 hand, I will not be answering many emails. Phone calls are better. Peter can do either, but email may be better for him. I will be providing my own updates from now on. The next will be around June 3rd, my four-year stroke anniversary. As you can imagine, I'm having a hard time emotionally right now, but I am very resilient and will get through this. I don't anticipate this affecting my rehab in any way. Thank you in advance for your support."

Going through this break-up was the hardest emotional experience I went through since my stay at Topanga Terrace. It was very unexpected, and since Peter had been the main source of information to my Caring Bridge followers, I thought it was necessary to let everyone know that Peter left me, and I would be taking over my own updates. Also, I wanted to stress that this loss would not hinder my rehab in any way. I am very stubborn, and I didn't want to pause or take a step back because of this change. While it was true that I didn't let it hinder my rehab, it was a very significant emotional period of my recovery.

By Sara Anderson— Jun 3, 2014 9:36pm

"Happy summer everyone!

Here in Wisconsin we certainly welcome summer after a particularly long, cold winter. I need to start this update by notifying you all that it will be my last. It also marks five years since my stroke! Since June 3rd, 2009, I have been working so hard to get back the things I know I certainly took for granted before my stroke. I think I have proven that I will not give up. I am doing all I can and will continue to do so. I encourage you to keep in touch, but the phone is much easier for me right now than email. I will also occasionally check caring bridge, so feel free to comment here too.

Instead of summarizing all my progress, I simply want to say thank you. This stroke has been devastating to me and my life, but the support I've received has made it much easier for me. We all have hard knocks in our life; the difference is our outlook and how we choose to react. I will try my best to continue to make this into a positive experience. This has been hard to do, but I'm determined to do it. The real reason that I'm even able to do this and continue to get better is my parents. I couldn't do this without them. They are the most amazing and selfless people I've ever met in my life. I aspire to be like them. Thank you Mom and Dad for everything! You are the best people in the world! I'm so proud to call you my parents! I love you so much!

I wish you all well and hope you enjoy your summers! Since the stroke, I've certainly had an aversion to photos. However, since this is my last journal update, I wanted to include a couple photos. (Look for the two photos in the Caring Bridge photo section.) Thank you to Mallory Beinborn for taking these photos and to Joni Beinborn for allowing me to fall in love with her horse, Peanut. I encourage you to visit Mallory's website at http://www.impulsephotographymb.com/EquinePhotos.htm to see a video of Peanut smiling. Just click on the arrow on Peanut's nose. It's so cute! Thank you again! love, Sara"

This post was of course very important to me because it was my last regular Caringbridge post. Peter's leaving definitely emphasized the fact that my parents hadn't, and I really wanted to thank and praise them both again for their magnificent and amazing efforts with me. I've always thanked them, and I will continue to do so forever. They truly deserve it. I also posted pictures of me for the first time since the stroke, which was a big deal, as I looked so different than I did before the stroke.

CHAPTER 11

First Stop on the Rehab Train: Topanga Terrace

OPANGA TERRACE IS a "convalescent home," a nicer name for a nursing home. Yes, here I was just twenty-seven years old and living in a nursing home. I even celebrated my twenty-eighth birthday in that nursing home. However, as awful as that may sound, I was treated like royalty. I think that was because I was so young, and the other patients were so much older. I stood out as someone the staff could relate to, so they treated me like one of their family. I made many dear friends there. Since most of the nurses were Hispanic, they spoke Spanish among themselves and also to some of the patients. I had studied Spanish as an undergraduate; however,

I had not used my Spanish for a very long time, so I was very much out of practice. Listening to them and eventually speaking a bit with them helped me get my Spanish listening fluency back while I was there. This, of course, was a kind of bonus rehab I experienced.

I arrived at Topanga Terrace when my mom returned to LA after finishing her radiation treatments for her breast cancer. She was told that the time had come for me to leave the hospital. When the hospital staff told my mom that I had to leave the hospital, she was stunned and wondered where they wanted me to go. I was only semi-awake and unable to speak or move. The social worker told her that patients in my disabled condition were always discharged as soon as possible after an "event." Obviously I could not go home, so I had to go to a "facility." The social worker gave my parents a list of possible living facilities and told them to pick one. They then visited and toured several nursing homes. Most seemed so dismal that they left my mother in tears at the end of the day. However, one of the facilities that they visited was in Topanga Canyon. They were given a tour by Deborah, the Admissions Director. My mother explained to Deborah that she was really having a hard time trying to envision her young daughter in a nursing home surrounded by so many elderly people. Deborah pointed out that there were only two patients to a room, and that she would try to get me next to one of the patio doors that were in each room. My mother found out later from the administrator that Topanga Terrace did not take patients as young as I was, but Deborah went to the administrator after they left and told her that they had to make an exception for me because "this mother has broken my heart."

When my friend Cary came for another visit and after reviewing the list of facilities, she joined my parents and Peter and went back to Topanga for a second visit. They all agreed it was definitely the brightest, cleanest, and friendliest facility they had seen. So, after almost a month in the ICU at Kaiser Sunset Hospital, where they had saved and stabilized my life, I was transported to Topanga Terrace to begin my recovery. I lived there from June 30 to September 30, 2009. Everyone thought it was extremely premature that I had to depart the ICU when I still needed so much help, but that was the hospital and the insurance provider's decision. My case worker felt I was ready to live in a convalescent home. There I would begin my long road of recovery and therapy.

On the afternoon of June 30, 2009, I was discharged from the hospital and loaded into an ambulance with two attendants, a driver, and my mother. My mother told the attendants that I had a very strong cough, and it was not necessary to constantly suction my trach. They made her sit in the front seat, so she rode with her head over her shoulder making sure that no one was too anxious to stick a suction tube down my trach on the very bumpy, excruciatingly long ambulance ride to Topanga Canyon. The chosen route took the ambulance within two blocks of my house. That knowledge brought my mother to tears, knowing that I was so close to my house and I couldn't go there. However, I didn't know it. We finally arrived at Topanga Terrace. My mom told the Topanga Terrace staff that very little trach suctioning was necessary. She was so pleased when they treated me very gently. I was settled in my room, my family was there with me and I was completely unaware of anything.

I want to start to describe the exceptional staff at Topanga, but I'll purposely leave out the therapists for now, as I describe their work in detail in a later chapter. When I arrived at Topanga,

June 30, 2009, I was totally paralyzed except for my little pinky finger on my right hand. I could lift that finger slightly. Everyone was very excited when I made this small movement. My parents would always mention this paralysis as a place of reference for people who were unfamiliar with my journey. The head of rehab at Topanga, Patti, said it was not enough movement for me to begin therapy at that time. The administrator, Sharon, came to visit with my parents and saw how upset my parents were that I would not be going to the therapy room. Sharon went to the head of rehab and told her that I would not just be left in my bed, but that I would be starting therapy as soon as possible. Every time I added a movement—a finger, a toe, a foot or an ankle, my mother rushed to find Patti, the head of rehab, to tell her how much I was improving, so I could get to go to the therapy room. Patti told my mom she could finally order therapy for me when I could move my whole hand.

We began with the same range of motion movements I had been doing before. When Dad was in the ICU with me he asked the nurses how he could help me when I couldn't move and they told him about the importance of range of motion exercises. My parents became therapists and spent all of their days moving parts of my body when the therapists were not in the room. They stretched my fingers, bent my wrists, arms, legs, ankles, feet, and toes. There was no conscious response from my muscles; yet I was in constant motion from their tag team effort all day, every day. They hoped that the less damaged half of my brain was receiving these cues and starting to relearn. I also need to add here that my parents didn't know it at the time, but this constant motion allowed me to recover so well later on. Many therapists commented on what good care I had after my stroke due to my range of motion, most likely from these constant stretches my parents did for me.

The staff treated me like a friend, a daughter, and a sister—every one of them! Everyone made me feel welcome. Anytime I wanted anything, they were there right away to help. After a handful of weeks, when I became more alert, they discovered that I understood Spanish because one night they saw the movie, *Titanic*, playing in Spanish on the TV in my room. They asked my parents why I was watching it. My parents explained I could understand it; I had studied Spanish and even lived in Spain for a semester. Word traveled fast and the nurses began to speak Spanish to me, which I could understand, even though I could no longer speak it fluently. Actually at that time, I couldn't even speak, period. My voice had not yet returned. Still, language comprehension was another great sign that my mind and memory were working clearly once more, as I could now understand both English and Spanish.

The CNAs, certified nursing assistants, were invaluable also. The nursing staff was wonderful. My mother had a visit with the head nurse, and the nurse told her that she had a meeting with the CNAs about me. Because I was nearly the same age as the nursing assistants, they wanted to know more about my case. I was in pain from my trach because I could not hold up my head. All of my muscles had no strength. It took two CNA's and my mom or dad to get me in a wheelchair. They could see my pain and sympathized with me. Consequently, their weekly meetings included more focus on my treatment. The supervisor said there was a marked difference in the CNA's and their care of all the patients because of me. Everyone benefited, and they became more attuned to their jobs and how they were helping everyone.

In my room there was a white dry-erase board where the staff would post the date and the names of the CNA's for the current shift. While I loved everyone there, I was especially excited whenever I saw the names, Lourdes and Karlenas (Karla), because they were so much fun. I liked them, and they really liked me too. They discovered that I really understood Spanish because they would tell jokes in Spanish to each other, and I would laugh at them. Mostly they would speak to me in English, but if other people were around, and they just wanted to speak to me, then they would speak Spanish because they knew I understood it.

Karla looked much younger than she actually was, so I thought she was in her teens. She was actually in her early twenties. She had a daughter, which surprised me because I thought she was so young. Karla also later learned that the boots to prevent foot drop bothered me, so she would come and remove them after my parents left. I was really grateful because it meant that I wouldn't have to wake up in pain and wait until my parents arrived in the morning to remove them. My favorite part of the day was when my dad would remove the boots even though I know how sad that sounds. My left Achilles tendon was really tight, so Mom applied hours of pressure to make my ankle flex. The boots may not have been so bad if they'd actually been taken off every four hours, which was the protocol, so my feet could rest for a bit.

Then there was Lourdes. I remember asking Lourdes if she had kids, and she replied in Spanish, "Yes, I have four headaches."

Also a CNA, Lourdes was genuinely nice and generous. Lourdes and I had many laughs together. Lourdes would also occasionally even paint my toenails and fingernails. Everyone was jealous because I got such preferential treatment from her. Many times people would ask me, "Who painted your nails?"

and I would just reply, "My friend."

I did not want to get Lourdes in trouble by mentioning her name, and I didn't want other patients to bother her to do the same things for them. Lourdes also gave me a set of three stuffed monkeys, and I still have them—a larger monkey, which I named "Lourdes" to remember her by and two smaller monkeys, which I named "Pedrito" and "Sarita." I gave "Sarita" to my patient friend, Emmanuel, so he would have something to remember me by. The generosity and kindness that Lourdes and Karla showed me will always stay with me. I am very grateful to have known them.

Raul also played a big role in my recovery. He was so nice. When I first arrived, Raul would come by my room to do a passive range of motion exercises on me before I was able to do therapy in the therapy room. Range of motion exercise is when someone repeatedly stretches each limb as far as it will go in each direction because I couldn't move the limbs myself. It's basically having someone do a full exercise routine on your body for you to keep your circulation going and prevent your body and joints from getting stiff or even frozen. The motions are also important to keep the brain and body communicating through each movement. My parents actually did range of motion exercises on me ever since the first day of the stroke. They would also ask whoever visited me to hold my hand or foot and move anything and everything to try to give my body more motion and more exercise. Sometimes all four of my limbs would be doing range of motion at the same time! My parents absolutely adored Raul, as did I. Whenever I would get a new bouquet of flowers in my room, from family and friends, Raul would say "Oh good, Sara. You got my flowers. (They weren't from Raul.) I hope Peter won't be upset!" My parents and I just laughed. My parents immediately liked Raul because he was so gentle with me, and he always had a smile on his face. I wish I could have gotten to know him better, but during the time he was assisting me, I had yet to regain much of my voice, so we couldn't talk.

Then there was Sandra. Sandra is another CNA, but she mostly worked the early shift. (Lourdes and Karla worked the night shift.) Sandra was often scheduled to work my room, which I enjoyed because I liked her as my CNA. She would come in and turn the TV station to VH1, so we could listen to music. I liked that too, but I couldn't move my finger to adjust the channel, so Sandra helped. Sandra would first get me ready for the day by giving me a bed bath, choosing what I would wear, then dressing me, and brushing my hair and sometimes even braiding it. If my hair looked different, the other nurses would ask me "Did Sandra brush your hair today?"

Sharon, the Administrator of Topanga Terrace, was remarkable to my family and to me. I was the same age as her daughter, so it was easy for her to empathize with my situation. She really went out of her way to ensure that I got good care. Even when I first arrived and couldn't move, she did everything she could to get me into physical therapy as quickly as possible. Sharon would visit me almost every day. When I could eat solid food, she often made me homemade mashed potatoes, which the nurses would warm up in the microwave. I am a pescatarian (I eat fish, but no other meat) and Topanga didn't have a large pescatarian or vegetarian menu, which limited my options, so the potatoes were a luxury. We always said she had a good name because it was the same as my mom's. I really don't know how to express here how wonderful she was to me and my family. Very simply, she was amazing.

One situation that Sharon was helpful with was my iPod. In

my Topanga room, my parents had my iPod set up to play my music for me. The doctors had told my parents that studies showed that any music that was familiar to me would help stimulate my brain, besides also giving me a bit of entertainment. It was supposed to play quietly as I slept. But one night, while I was sleeping, the iPod was stolen. I was still paralyzed at that stage, I couldn't move, so someone just came into my room, and stole it. It was a terrible thing to do. Sharon recognized how terrible it was and that it reflected badly on Topanga Terrace. She said we could buy a new iPod, and she would reimburse us. Prior to that, she also offered a $300 cash reward for my original iPod, no questions asked, but it was never returned. The doctor who cared for my trach even added another cash reward of $300 for the return of the iPod. My parents were shocked that anyone would steal from a paralyzed girl. Sharon let my brother purchase a new one for me.

Speaking of people having the same names as my parents, it is also fitting to acknowledge Gary "line 101." I created the "line 101" because at Topanga there would be calls for Gary, and they would always page him as "Gary, line 101." Gary is the head of respiratory at Topanga. At the time I had a tracheotomy in my throat, so I saw Gary often. We all hated the trach, as it was uncomfortable for me when moving around, caused me to cough and feel irritated. But the trach was needed until the staff felt I could breathe without choking. My mom thought the trach was becoming increasingly unnecessary, so she was always asking Gary when it could be removed. A doctor came on Sunday mornings to check the status of everyone's trach. My mother cornered him every week and pleaded with him to downsize or remove the tube. Finally the trach was downsized to a smaller size. My friend Lucienne was visiting when Gary came in to insert the smaller trach. She held my hands while the large tube was removed and the smaller one was inserted. All went well. My mother then started her crusade to have that trach removed. She was always advocating for me, and she knew my swallowing reflex was very strong. Finally the doctor agreed to let me leave Topanga one afternoon and go to another hospital for a swallowing test. I had to go in an ambulance because of the trach. At the hospital, I had to sit in front of an x-ray machine while a doctor fed me different foods with different textures. Mom was able to sit with the x-ray technician to watch my swallowing progress.

The test went well, so the doctor said that the trach could be capped for brief periods to check my breathing. Around this time I was in the therapy room and I made a sound that I'm told sounded like a duck quacking. This only happened once and it was only air escaping around the trach but my parents were just happy to hear any sound. I broke into tears. My emotions were so raw and on edge. Up to this point in time, I had not been able to speak. My mom put her face to mine to say, "I love you, Sara. Can you say 'Mom?'" I was crying and she was crying but somehow I whispered "Hi Mom."

It brought my mom so much joy to hear this! With the cap on the trach, I was forced to fully breathe on my own. Before they capped it the first time, they told me that it might be a little scary because I wasn't used to breathing through my nose and mouth; however, I didn't notice any difference at all. I handled the cap well, but I had to keep the trach "capped," or closed for twenty-four hours before the doctor would agree to its complete removal. In fact, I didn't have any difficulty with it being capped whatsoever. Finally, the trach was removed from my throat in early August, after nearly two months of living with it. They removed the trach by just pulling it out of my neck, and it wasn't painful. I didn't even have to go to the hospital to have it removed surgically.

As soon as the trach was removed, my mom started lobbying for the removal of the G-tube, or feeding tube, that I had in my stomach. I had finally gained better control of my facial muscles, and I was able to open my mouth, and swallow soft foods. It was so exciting to taste food and drink again. After having liquid food, vitamins and water just run through a tube directly into my stomach, eating and drinking made me feel really more "normal" again.

I was very thirsty from the tracheotomy. When I had the trach and G-tube, I wasn't allowed to eat or drink anything, for fear I would choke. So you can imagine how thirsty I was when I wasn't allowed to drink. Sometimes Mom would ask the nurses to give me an extra "drink" through my G-tube, and they would do so by filling a syringe up with water and squirting it into the G-tube, a plastic tube that was surgically inserted into my stomach. I know this procedure doesn't sound like much of a "drink," but I could feel the water entering my body through the G-tube and re-hydrating me, and it did provide some relief. I also looked forward to the nurses brushing my teeth nightly because I could swallow little drops of water then. I remember one night that Karla, the CNA, discovered that I wanted water, so she filled a glass with water and said to me in Spanish "Slowly, be careful! Really, this scares me." I sipped the water fine and was so thankful to her for the drink. Later on, when I was finally able to drink, I often asked for juice for some more taste. Prior to the stroke I never would have chosen juice due to its high sugar and calorie content. Dad made so many trips from my room to the kitchen of Topanga Terrace that he joked that I should have a conveyer belt installed from my room to the kitchen. I just wanted something to drink, and the juice was very quenching. I later heard from other patients that had tracheotomies that they too were just as thirsty.

When the G-Tube was finally removed, I was finally "un-hooked," which had been my mom's foremost mission. The food tube in my stomach, the trach in my throat, and the IV's in both arms were now gone. When it was agreed that the G-Tube could be removed, my parents and I wanted to know how they were going to get it out of my stomach. A doctor said that they just hold you down and yank it out. My mom, however, felt that I had suffered enough and let it be known that there wasn't going to be any pain involved and that I would be asleep during the brief procedure. She talked to a woman doctor at Topanga, and the doctor was very understanding and agreed to set my appointment with a doctor at the hospital whom she felt was also very understanding.

Our trip to the hospital this time was in my car. It wasn't easy since we had to put the wheelchair in the trunk, but my parents managed it, and so I took my first ride in my car since my stroke. I just wanted to adjust the radio stations and look in the glove compartment and touch everything I could to see how much I remembered. It was all familiar. It was so emotional that finally I just started to cry. It had just been so long since I had seen my car. At the hospital, my mother stood firm, saying that I would be put to sleep for the procedure. The doctor finally agreed and the permission slips were signed.

It was only a five-minute procedure, but I was so happy that I didn't have to feel any unnecessary pain. I woke up, the hated tube was gone, and I realized I was finally "wireless." Compared to the first couple of weeks after the stroke, which I had no memory of, I had improved so much that I felt I was almost "too awake" now. I was too conscious and recognizing all of the challenges I had to conquer in order to get better. I was becoming too aware of everything. Still, I wanted to return to the state of being able to do therapy and improve, but not really be too conscious. I would often tell Mom, "I think I'm too awake now!"

Neuroplasticity is the ability of the brain to relearn skills that another part of the brain is suddenly unable to do. My stroke severely affected my balance, motor skills, and coordination centers in the back and the right side of my brain. In fact, the truth of the matter is that much of the right side of my cerebellum was killed by the stroke. However, the part of my brain that held my memory was unaffected, so I knew what I wanted my body to do. It was just that the damaged parts of the right side of my brain were unable to carry out any of my commands.

On June 30, twenty-six days after my stroke, I was still almost totally paralyzed. I had to start from scratch and relearn how to move every part of my body. In the hospital, the doctors would command, "Squeeze my hand," or "Wiggle your toes." Initially, I could respond, but the longer that I lay in my bed, the weaker my response would be. Undeterred, my parents believed that I would beat the odds, so they continually moved me, even when I couldn't respond. They had been educated by the doctors about neuroplasticity and the fact that the brain is an amazing organ that can actually "rewire" itself. In other words, the undamaged part of a brain can relearn everything that the damaged part of that same brain initially knew. Every time a movement is repeated, the brain knows and tries to form a link to the movement. Slowly, ever so slowly, I was able to move all of the fingers on my right hand and my right ankle started moving back and forth.

Brain injured patients need lots of sleep, and it is during that sleep that the brain considers all of the movements that occurred during the day and builds a little wire link to those movements. However, we later believed the body needed more than a little wire—it needed a thick wire, almost like a cable. Acquiring that cable requires repetition of a movement, not just one time, not a hundred times, but many thousands of times. Stubbornness, determination, and dedication to overcome hopelessness in one's lack of movement is the key to recovering that movement freely. Sometimes a stroke victim just wants to give up and live with the deficits. However, I wasn't like that. Come hell or high water I was going to recover. I wasn't going to settle for anything less than pretty damn near perfect.

One night my mom was holding my left hand when my arm and the hand went rigid. My mom kept massaging it until it finally relaxed. She checked with the therapist the next day and was told that I had "tone." When you see brain injured patients sometimes, you may notice that their arms are curled up close to their chest and just don't want to relax into a normal position. That is what tone or spasticity can do to a person who lacks control of their body. The therapist told my mother that if this happened again, to massage my arm and hand until the spastic seizure let go and then stretch my hand back to a 90 degree angle to stretch out my forearm muscle and hold it in that position as long as possible. From that point on, my mother stretched that muscle several times an hour, even when it did not spasm. She wanted to keep that muscle loose. My mother protected my arm from curling simply by constantly stretching and moving my body. Later, we learned that a simple, (painless) brace would have prevented this problem, and I should have had it put on almost immediately after the stroke. The body likes to curl up after a stroke and the muscles get abnormally shorter, so wearing a simple brace to keep the hand flat while you sleep is painless and will prevent this from happening and give you a nice, stretched out flat hand.

I slept a lot more after the stroke. At first, I would sleep a lot during the day and also at night. But then as I became more alert, I no longer slept much through the day. Before the stroke, I didn't take any naps. I never had been a good nap person. The same became true after the stroke once I became alert enough. The doctors prescribed some medicine to help keep me conscious. They wanted me alert and moving. However at night I found I did sleep much more. I almost always got at least ten hours of good sleep. Sometimes, I slept nearly twelve hours. I was never sleepy during the day, but I definitely didn't feel like I was getting too much sleep either. I had heard that lengthy sleeping was normal, and that patients slept more during their recovery as well, so I didn't think anything abnormal about wanting a lot of sleep to help my brain heal. While sleeping, the brain is still working and processing the movements that occurred during the previous day. As time progressed and after several years in Wisconsin, I gradually required less sleep than my usual twelve hours. I recognized that change when I naturally started waking up earlier on my own. I remember once telling my parents when they tried to wake me that I needed to sleep more because my brain wasn't done rewiring. That excuse didn't work, but I thought it was clever.

There were many different characters and personalities at Topanga Terrace; however, there was one man we found rather amusing. We would go to the therapy room, and this older gentleman was often in there at the same time. He was a retired doctor, who was also a patient, let's just all him "the doctor." While these were difficult days in the early stages of my recovery, the doctor provided some comic relief for us. He was there because he suffered from Alzheimer's disease. While there is nothing funny about Alzheimer's disease, the doctor had a very colorful personality and vocabulary, and he always challenged everyone around him.

As I was doing my therapy one day, I heard him ask his therapist, "Why are you doing these maneuvers on me?" To us, it was very funny, but to the therapists, the doctor was just obnoxious. I also remember him repeatedly calling his therapist "Omar" or "Abraham," when his name was actually Raj. Then one day I entered the therapy room, and I was placed on a therapy mat. The doctor saw me and asked very loudly, "What is that woman doing on my mat? Doesn't she know it's reserved for me?"

My parents and I thought the doctor was so funny, and laughing was good for us during that time. Dad would also try to lift my spirits by telling me that "the worst is over" and "the biggest thing you have going for you is your age." The latter comment he would say because it's the elderly who suffer from strokes more frequently, so I definitely had age on my side to motivate me to get better. Mom once said people who have strokes are typically over sixty years of age. If they could do the therapy, then I should be able to shine at it. She knew that pre-stroke, I went to the gym five days a week and had a definite mindset to exercise. I wasn't afraid to sweat and work hard. I also knew I should be able to tolerate the rigorous therapy schedule because of my young age and fitness level.

I knew I had so much life left ahead of me that I couldn't give up like some other stroke patients who felt that the endless repeating exercises were too much. I knew I had to stay focused and push myself toward daily improvement, as I would not be satisfied otherwise. So from the start, I was determined to stay committed to daily therapy despite progress being excruciatingly slow. I realized how much of life I still had ahead of me. It was always very helpful to hear positive words of encouragement from those around me because it was really a very scary time for me. When I was scared, I would just think of Jen, who also suffered a stroke and yet had recovered so well. I would also remember the calm feeling my mom had on the plane coming to see me immediately after the stroke. I thought that it was a good sign that I would ultimately be okay.

CHAPTER 12

New Friends and Roommates

OPANGA WAS INVALUABLE to me in many ways because I made lifelong friends there. Emmanuel is definitely one of them. Emmanuel is older than me by several decades, and he was at Topanga to do physical therapy for walking; he had to have one of his legs amputated due to poor circulation, a condition that may have started for him while he was serving in WWII. He would voluntarily increase the resistance on any machine he used, hoping it would get him better faster. I liked Emmanuel even before I knew him because my mom said he reminded her of her dad, my Grandpa Sieber. I would have loved him anyway for his energy, his spirit, and his kindness, but that comparison made our connection immediate. Emmanuel's wife, Josie, is just as sweet. Josie was with Emmanuel every day, and she loved me and my family just like Emmanuel did. Emmanuel would always call me his "angel" and we would wave to each other and give the thumbs up sign to each other when our wheelchairs passed in the hallway or whenever we were in the therapy room at the same time. He was very encouraging and a great role model for me to say the least. He would take my hand and say, "We will learn to walk together."

When I was getting ready to leave Topanga, I went and found Emmanuel and gave him one of the little monkeys that Lourdes had given me. I had named it "Sarita." He put it sitting on his nightstand. When I talked to Emmanuel and Josie today by phone after returning to Wisconsin, he often mentioned "Sarita," so I'm glad that little monkey went to a good home. Emmanuel has now received a prosthetic leg and walks with it, and he has gotten his driver's license back, so his hard work really paid off in the end.

Windi is another friend. She was a younger patient like me at Topanga, so it was nice to have her company. Windi has such a sad story. At the time of her accident, she was married, with two children and pregnant with her third. On her daughter's birthday, she was driving to pick something up for the party, and a car hit her on the freeway by pulling ahead of her and then slamming on the brakes and sending her crashing. Her kids in the backseat were okay, but Windi broke her back. It left her a paraplegic for life. The Jaws of Life had to be used get her out of the car. She fought to remain conscious long enough to tell the rescuers that she was pregnant. Windi named the little girl she was carrying at the time Casey after her sister who had tragically passed away in a different accident when they both were younger. Sadly, Windi's husband left her and took their kids soon after the accident because he didn't want to deal with having a paralyzed wife. As scary as that story is for anyone to imagine, Windi maintained a great positive attitude and was always very thoughtful and generous to everyone. Windi would roll her wheelchair into my room at Topanga almost every night even before I was able to speak.

Dad, Aunt Marilyn, Sara, Mom at Topanga Terrace

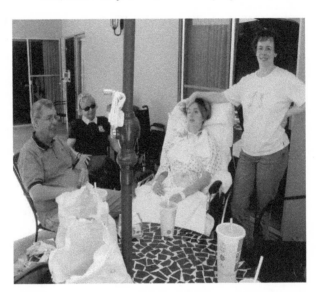

You can imagine just how hard it is to get to know someone when you can't even hold a conversation with anyone. However, while I lay in my bed, Windi would always talk, and I would listen. Windi would often read me magazines, including my horoscope, from the newspaper. My dad reads the newspaper every day and would leave the horoscope section for Windi because he knew how much she liked it. She would talk about lighthearted topics and girly topics to distract the two of us from our reality for a bit.

Windi was definitely cheering me to recover, and we often talked by phone after I returned to Wisconsin.

My roommates at Topanga were also noteworthy. First there was Geri, who I don't remember at all, as during my first few weeks at Topanga I was largely unconscious. Justa was my next roommate. Justa came from Cuba, and she is bilingual. Her daughter and granddaughter, both named Andrea, would visit late at night to accommodate the mother's work schedule. Justa was in her late seventies, and she was staying in Topanga because someone had tried to break into her house early one morning and she got tangled in the sheets and fell down as she was trying to get to the phone to call the police. She was seriously injured and had to have a trach, but she was also trying to get better and leave.

Justa would often be hooked up to breathing machines that would beep all the time whenever her breathing became labored and my parents always checked to make sure she was okay. She always was. Justa and I shared a TV in the room, and she always wanted to watch baseball for some reason. At that time, I wasn't a fan of baseball; however, now I consider myself a solid Milwaukee Brewers fan. I thought it was so odd that she loved watching it. I ended up watching a lot of the Dodgers' season that summer. At that stage, however, I couldn't even press the button to change the channel even if I wanted to. I never got to know Justa because I couldn't speak while she was my roommate. She was always concerned for me though, and she told my parents that she prayed for me always.

One time she had a visitor who came to see her, and her visitor also talked to me. After asking my mom if she could touch me, she sat at the end of my bed and talked to my mother and rubbed my motionless left foot. A week or so later Justa's daughter asked to talk to my mother in private. She wanted to know if my mom remembered this woman's visit. She told her she did.

Justa's daughter told her this woman had spoken to a friend of hers who was a clairvoyant. The psychic interrupted their conversation and told her she had recently touched a young woman with a wounded left leg. Justa's friend told her that she had been at the nursing home visiting her friend, Justa, and had spoken to her roommate. The clairvoyant told her that the young girl's leg would recover and she would walk again and she would be able to return to her previous profession. Andrea told my mom that when her friend told her this story it gave her the "shivers" but she just wanted my mom to know about it. My mom didn't tell me this story at the time it happened but shared the story with my friend Reka. They agreed to keep the story to themselves and await the outcome of my therapy. Later, when Mom told me the story, I loved it, especially how it was from a woman who never met me, yet she was foretelling a positive feeling about my full recovery. I thought it was very interesting.

Rosaline was my next roommate, but only for a few days. Rosaline was in her seventies, and I don't even remember why she was in Topanga. She wasn't my favorite roommate. I don't mean to be rude or disrespectful, but she was difficult to share a room with. All day and all night she would scream "No!" "Help me!" "My back!" The staff would come right away, but as soon as they would leave she would yell the same way again. The staff became desensitized to her call because she would do the same thing over and over again. They didn't know how to help her. As a result, I didn't get much rest while Rosy was my roommate. I couldn't speak, and she wouldn't be quiet. We were quite the opposites.

My parents and Sharon, the administrator, recognized the

problem and reassigned me to another room as soon as possible. My parents were very worried that my lack of sleep would negatively affect my focus and energy during my therapy. That didn't happen though because I switched rooms so quickly. My last roommate was Peggy. I really liked Peggy, as did my parents. Peggy was in her sixties. She was getting dizzy spells and falling from being off balance. She had recently fallen, hit her head, and hurt her wrist and shoulder, so she was brought to Topanga to be evaluated and do therapy to get stronger before returning home. Peggy was very quiet and easy to share a room with. I enjoyed having her as a roommate. She felt bad for me because I was so young. She told my parents that during the time she spent with me she noticed my behavior was beginning to change. She thought I was like a small child when she came, but when I left, she said I was almost a teenager again.

I don't remember much about June or July, 2009, but I do remember the pattern of my days. First, I would wake up and those awful boots would be on my feet and my legs would be in a lot of pain, especially the left leg. After waking in the morning, I would always try to press the help button, but I couldn't press it. They later resolved the issue by giving me a more sensitive very large button to push if I ever needed anything. However, once I could press the button in the morning, the nurses would come, but I couldn't speak to tell them to "please remove the boots." The boots were supposed to be four hours off and four hours on, but I don't ever remember the nurses taking them off. So I would have to wait until my parents arrived around 8 a.m. Then they would take the boots off my feet. Immediately, I was very relieved. Then, we would go to physical therapy for a full workout, then back to my room. Then I would have my peanut butter and jelly sandwich and fruit plate for lunch, then more lengthy therapy again. After that, we would go back to my room and watch old reruns of *I Love Lucy* and *Hawaii Five-O*. My parents thought maybe I would recognize details from the show since I had lived in Hawaii. My parents would leave between 7:00 and 8:00 p.m. and Windi would come and visit.

CHAPTER 13

What's Happening to Me?

MY BROTHER, BRIAN, and his wife, Melanie, made a second trip to LA to spend a week with me. It was to be a great time because my sister, Lisa, and my niece and nephews were also supposed to come the same week. However, one day after Brian and Melanie arrived, tragedy struck again. On August 24, my grandpa Sieber died. My parents talked to me after therapy, and my mom told me that her father, my grandpa, Robert Charles Sieber, had passed away that morning. How awful! So in less than a year, my mom had been diagnosed with breast cancer, I had had a stroke and my Grandpa had died. Mom telling me about Grandpa was the worst time emotionally for me during my journey post-stroke.

First of all, I didn't believe it was real. I told my parents later that I thought I was just stuck in some kind of a nightmare. Nothing seemed real, and I was so confused and scared. I asked everyone around me how to wake up from a nightmare. When offered, I used an alphabet board to spell out the phrase, "Wake me up." My mom kept telling me that I was awake, but I didn't believe her.

The only other times I haven't been able to move or scream have been in my own nightmares, so maybe this time was no different. Everything that Mom had told me about having a stroke seemed absurd because I was so young and healthy. So at the time I did not believe it was possible. Again, I was very ignorant about strokes. What I did know was that elderly people suffered from strokes. But I was in my twenties! My parents thought I meant a metaphorical nightmare, which it absolutely was, but I really meant it felt like a literal nightmare. I felt trapped in an endless nightmare, and I could not wake myself up. I was very scared and terribly confused. My parents even brought me stories from the Internet about other young women who had suffered strokes. Now, when I read them, they completely make sense because I have a similar tale. But at the time, none of it made sense and hearing those stories wasn't what I wanted.

I know it sounds crazy, but I was certain I was trapped in a nightmare, and hopefully, I would just wake up and everything would be the same again. For many days, I would open my eyes, hoping I would "wake up." I was always disappointed when everything was the same, and I would have to go through another long day of arduous therapy. I tried to do everything I could to make the nightmare end. I tried to remember previous nightmares and think about how they ended. I recalled in one of my nightmares, I was able to act inappropriately or out of character and it ended. When I tried this "trick" by saying things or acting out of character to the nurses or therapists, of course it didn't work. It just left me embarrassed. I felt very bad about acting out because it was so out of character for me, but then I realized that I had to give myself a bit of a break and forgive myself because everything in my life was so odd, and I was just desperate to get back to normal. I still don't think that my "nightmare" hypothesis is that silly when I was trying to analyze and understand what was going on. The scariest part for me, however, when I reflect back on this time was the confusion I experienced then. I didn't understand what was happening to me, which was why I was trying to find anything anywhere that could explain what was happening to me. It was truly like living a real nightmare.

I do remember having one dream in particular around that time. I dreamt that I was in Topanga Terrace, but Topanga Terrace was actually the house of my mom's neighbor, Elna, in Wisconsin. Elna's house is right next to my mom's house, which is the house where I grew up. I got out of bed and ran to my own house and lay down in my own bed. I loved this dream for obvious reasons, and I was very disappointed when I had to realize later that it wasn't reality. However, for that dream, I was able to have a dream within a dream because at that time I was very sure I was really trapped in a dream in my own life. It actually made me feel like the dream was a good sign, telling me that I wasn't dreaming after all because at the time I believed you can't ever have a dream within a dream. So therefore, none of any of it could be real and I'd soon wake up. Just thinking this brought me some much-needed relief.

As I said, my brother Brian and my sister-in-law Melanie were with me at this time. It was comforting for me because my mom had to return to Wisconsin for my Grandpa's funeral. Of course Brian and I wanted to mourn our Grandpa at the funeral, but I was not well enough to travel, and it was very difficult for Brian and Melanie to find a last-minute flight back to Wisconsin, as they had just arrived to see me in California. My mom just said "Grandpa would want them to stay with me." So that's what they did. While Mom returned to Wisconsin to do one of the hardest things in her life, Brian and Melanie spent a lot of time at my bedside. I was very scared during this time because of my nightmare theory.

Struggling with the thought of being trapped forever in a literal nightmare, I tried to remember my past nightmares and what I did to end them. Sometimes I have had nightmares where I would die, and those would startle me, and I would kind of jump when I awakened. So I thought that maybe now I would have to try to kill myself in the dream I thought I was having in real life, so hopefully I could "wake up" and be fine again. That was scary for me, especially because everything seemed so real. Physically, the only way I could imagine that reality was to fall out of my wheelchair and land just right. I thought this best-case scenario of falling was I would "wake up" and that experience would just be one of my former dreams that was so real. However, being an empathetic person, I would consider those therapists who were working with me, and I would never risk getting them in trouble by falling out of my wheelchair, just in case I was wrong about this being a dream and it was actually reality. I didn't want to get anyone in trouble by getting hurt.

I also didn't mind when the nursing staff physically moved me around my bed or washed and dressed me because I wanted to be jolted awake. Other times when I was hoping to be awakened was when my hair was brushed in the morning or when they used electrode therapy on me and let electrical current run through my body to stimulate my nerves and muscles. I hoped this stimulation would awaken me from my real dream that wasn't a dream at all.

Mom would show me an alphabet board because I could spell, but not speak. I would often spell "wake me up." Mom would always say, "Sara, you're not sleeping." Then, I thought about that statement and realized that you only get one chance at "reality." I even thought maybe the dream was somehow watching me (I know, that sounds totally crazy). I felt scared and alone and confused. It was unsettling to say the least. Then I began to believe that someone was in charge of the dream, so I needed to figure out who it was in order to be "released." I was already close to the people in charge at Topanga; Sharon, the administrator, was the head of Topanga and visited me daily. Patti was my physical therapist and the head of Topanga rehab. I tried to say "yes" when I meant to say "no" and vice versa, to see if the dream was reading my mind. It was another attempt to end the nightmare. For example, my parents were kind enough to request a room with a patio entrance as they knew I love to be outdoors, yet whenever they asked me if I wanted to sit out on that patio I would always say "no," although of course I meant "yes"! Who wouldn't want to be outside on a nice day? Again, this was my way to see if my life dream could read my mind and one more attempt to "wake up." I regretted this action later when I realized that I was not trapped in a dream at all. I was living my own reality.

Feeling suicidal in "the dream" felt too real and scary for me even to consider, so I thought maybe I should wait and finish the dream. Thank goodness I did that and stopped thinking this way. When Mom returned, I was able to talk to her, and then I felt like I wasn't stuck in a dream anymore. It felt so comforting not to feel trapped in a dream. It wasn't anything she said. I just felt calmed after talking to her. Maybe it was her leaving like she had to do for Grandpa's funeral and her promise to be back in a couple of days that was the key to waking me up. I remember thinking about whether or not this idea was even slightly feasible. Could all these people be visiting me? Could I actually be totally paralyzed? Could my parents really be living with Peter for this long in California? While all these questions were extremely far fetched, it WAS possible. Then I started to ask myself, "What's the last thing I remember?" I remembered going to the clinic, but I didn't remember leaving. It made sense because that's where my mom's story began. So maybe this ridiculous, yet consistent, story about the stroke was true!

Later, during the same period, I knew that while I didn't want to be stuck in a nightmare, I also thought that the nightmare theory, while terrifying, was the best option. I thought I could just "wake up" and resume my life as it was before the stroke. Unfortunately that wasn't the case. I didn't really understand the severity of the situation and all the hard work that lay ahead of me. I had to learn about it and accept what was happening to me and then dig deep inside to find the motivation to work hard for several years to try to reclaim my life.

While my recovery was lengthy and very difficult, I remained determined to try my best, especially after seeing how hard everyone around me was fighting for me. I found it only fair to fight just as hard for them. I also began to cry a lot during this time. At first I didn't mind crying because I remembered a nightmare that I had once that ended when I cried and I woke up. However, I continued to cry uncontrollably, which prompted the doctors to prescribe me an anti-depressant. I didn't like this direction because I was never on any anti-depressants before the stroke. I have always had a happy demeanor, and my stroke was most likely caused by a medication so I wasn't real excited to be told to take more medication. However, it did help me. I stopped crying so much. I later learned that my depression was most likely misdiagnosed, and I was more likely suffering from pseudobulbar affect (PBA). This condition offers a neurological reason for inappropriate periods of crying. It would explain my sometimes inappropriate bouts of crying. Yet by the time the real cause was identified, I was in no way willing to take more medication. I also felt like time was helping me improve by the time PBA was identified. When I saw my mother again, I knew that everything was real, and that all that she had told me about what had happened to me was true. Prior to that realization, I was terrified. Sometimes you just need your Mom, I guess. I certainly needed her then.

It was too bad for Brian and Melanie though, since I was acting awfully weird whenever they visited. I would ask them to "Google how to get out of a nightmare and print the results to show me." I wanted a checklist of actions to use to "escape." I tried everything I could think of. I also asked Brian and Melanie to think of their own nightmares and what they did to get out of them, and then make me a checklist, which they did. The theme of their lists more or less told me to "take control." I had them post the lists on the walls in my room. I even told Windi one night when she visited that I thought everything was all a dream. Brian also asked each of my therapists what I needed to do to get out of Topanga faster. Then he and Melanie made a checklist about each of my therapies (physical, occupational and speech) and those lists were hung in my room too. Once I didn't feel I was stuck in a dream anymore, that what was happening to me really was reality, I started to think about everything I knew that had happened. When my brother, Brian, visited he said some really nice things to me and I remembered them and also questioned if they were real. I thought his visit was so nice, and I was happy to believe it was real.

If I had realized all that had to be done to try to help me, a nightmare would have actually been the best option, since I could just wake up and be normal again. Yet I was relieved to know my life was real because at least I understood reality; I didn't understand my "nightmare." Because I didn't understand my current reality either, a stroke reality was less scary to me. Also, I asked myself, am I okay being a stroke survivor forever? I accepted this view before I knew what it meant. Later, I realized that I would always be tied to older people, since that is the population that usually suffers from stroke. I was twenty-seven when I suffered this debilitating stroke. Also, now people often believe I represent ALL strokes. As much as I hated the "all strokes are different" response from doctors and therapists, it is so true.

Often people want to tell me about a family member or friend who suffered a stroke, but it's not very relatable because of the fact that all strokes are different. I can relate to the struggle and slowness, but that's about all. A stroke affects your brain and, therefore, different parts of your body, as opposed to a broken leg, for example, which may affect many people more similarly. If I had been correctly diagnosed initially at the hospital, I knew I would have had a very different outcome and perhaps even a minimal recovery time. However, I never got the chance to receive the clot-busting drug that could have saved my brain and let me have an easier recovery. Regardless, I'm very proud to be a stroke survivor.

I even remember talking to my mom around this time when I was starting to believe my stroke was real. I acknowledged all that she had been through and all she had done for me and then said, "You deserve the mother of the year award!" I still believe that. Similarly, Dad deserves the "father of the year" award. It's remarkable how much my parents selflessly did for me. I also remember trying to invoke "Mom powers." I was not a mother, so I didn't know if this power existed, but I thought it was worth a shot, so I told her "I can't move the left side of my body." I was hoping she would use her "Mom powers" to fix everything for me immediately. Of course, she didn't have any "special" powers, but as I mentioned, I believe she is without a doubt the best mother in the world. I believe her love and support were and still are as valuable as any "Mom powers" I was curious about and hoped she had at that time.

I got tired of constantly hearing the word "progress" because I heard it all the time, and I didn't think it was accurate for me. I never felt or saw progress in the early days and beyond due to my incredibly high standards for recovery. I figured if I wasn't exactly again how I had been pre-stroke, then I wasn't making progress. I never considered my paralysis months earlier and compared it to where I was now. This mentality followed me for way too long. When I would go to therapy from my room to the rehab room at Topanga Terrace shortly after my stroke, we always met someone who would stop us and comment on all the "progress" I had made. However, I would tell my mom after we left, "I don't know them!"

She would just say "You met them when we first arrived." I simply had and still have no memory of when I first arrived at Topanga Terrace.

Shortly after my mom returned and Brian and Melanie left,

I learned I would soon be moving to Northridge Hospital. I asked everyone at Topanga what they thought of Northridge and everyone (including the CNAs and the therapists) said their rehab program had a great reputation. Upon hearing that, I wanted to go there because everyone who knew the program gave it a big thumbs up.

Dr. Pigeon, the Rehab Director at Northridge Hospital, visited Topanga Terrace every week to observe potential patients that could graduate and go to Northridge Hospital. Dr. Pigeon is very nice and he would watch me in therapy and talk to my therapists. He encouraged me to join the program at Northridge. He thought I was ready for the next level of rehabilitation. So after one month in the Kaiser ICU and three months at Topanga Terrace nursing home, Northridge Hospital is where my journey continued.

CHAPTER 14

Second Stop: Northridge Hospital

HE MOVE TO Northridge Hospital was bittersweet because we had spent so much time at Topanga where we were treated so well and we had made so many friends. We said our goodbyes, which were very emotional because we knew how much everyone had helped bring me back to consciousness and restart my life. Leaving Topanga felt like the end of an era, a period of my life, but it was also a happy moment because I knew I was graduating to the next level of rehabilitation and recovery. My stroke happened June 3, 2009. I moved to Topanga Terrace on June 30, 2009. I moved to Northridge Hospital on September 30, 2009. My parents and I were all very excited to have me move to Northridge Hospital because of the strong therapy reputation it had. The hospital is supposed to be the best in the region for stroke rehabilitation. When I left Northridge, I was still kind of disappointed in my progress. I had arrived in a wheelchair, and I left in a wheelchair. I thought I would be able to walk unassisted. Of course, I always had very unrealistic expectations.

I have several memories of my first evening at Northridge. On that first evening, we "checked in" and they gave me a new hospital bracelet that displayed my name, address, phone number, etc. I wondered how long it would be wrapped around my wrist. Then we went up to my floor, and they placed me in a holding room, which had six beds. I was the only patient there. It was called the "Big Room." I was promised I would be moved into my own private room the next day, and I was excited about that. At Topanga, I always had a roommate. I enjoyed having a roommate. In the early months of my recovery, it was better for me to have a roommate, as I still had the trach and couldn't talk and couldn't move much. However, I had been in hospitals for several months now, so I was also looking forward to a bit more privacy. My roommates could keep an eye on me if I signaled that I had any discomfort or needs. But now because I was more alert, a bit more stable, and had others around me all the time during the day (my parents, the nurses or therapists), a private room at Northridge sounded very appealing.

My first meal at Northridge was a little difficult. At Northridge they have a food menu. It lets you choose what you want to eat. However, on that first night, the kitchen just sent a food tray to my room and hoped it would be okay. It wasn't. It was beef tips, and I don't eat meat. The kitchen was able to give me a different meal though, and Dad gladly ate the mistake. Having a menu at Northridge that included a handful of vegetarian options (veggie stir fry, veggie lasagna, veggie soups, etc.) was very welcomed, after the very limited menu I had had at Topanga.

I also remember a nurse named Tori, who came to check on me that first night. She gave me a little test to check my memory. She said, "I'm going to say three words and you need to remember them, because I'll ask you for them again in a minute." "Okay," I said, unworried. "White. Volkswagen. Turtle."

We then talked for a bit, and a minute later she asked me "Sara, what were the three words I asked you to remember?" "White. Volkswagen. Turtle," I said.

I knew I had a good memory, and I didn't mind showing that off. Even when I saw Tori weeks later, I would still repeat those three words to prove that I could still remember them. She always gave me a big smile back. That first night she also told me, "Dr. Pigeon will be here very early tomorrow morning." I found out she wasn't kidding. Dr. Pigeon arrived around 6 a.m. the next day. I learned he visited his patients every day very early just like that. He would always call me by my first and last name, not just "Sara." I thought that was kind of cute.

That first morning he spoke to me about the program at Northridge and wanted to make sure that I was comfortable in my new environment. While everything was new, everyone seemed nice, and I was comfortable. I was happy to have my own room, which was much quieter. Plus, I could control the television, so I could watch what I wanted to when my long day of therapy was done.

Every morning at Northridge, they give you a printed schedule for your daily therapy in PT, OT and Speech. My therapies the first day were general evaluations. They wanted to test what level I was at. In PT, they had me kneel on a mat, and the therapists began pushing on me from all directions, seeing if I could maintain my balance. I was pretty good at right and left, but it was very challenging to resist being pushed forward and backward. From there, my daily schedule continued with sessions of PT, OT and Speech. I spent many hours practicing and relearning all my movements and daily functions. While I was regaining some basic movement, I still had to be assisted with washing, dressing, eating, walking, etc. Thankfully, my arms and legs were moving, my left slower than my right, and I could communicate directly, but only with a weak voice.

One of the things I really liked immediately about Northridge was that I was given an "estimated discharge date." We were told that the hospital would look to discharge me at the beginning of November. I checked in on September 30, so compared to my three months at Topanga (June 30–September 30), five weeks at Northridge didn't sound like that long a time. Plus, I really didn't want to keep my parents away from Wisconsin during the upcoming holidays. I was excited to be able to count down my days. I knew Northridge would be my last hospital stop before going home. Of course, I also thought I would be completely better when I was discharged. After six months of living hospital life, nothing sounded better than enjoying the comforts of home. However, my attitude would later change and I would I hope I could lengthen my stay to avoid going home in a wheelchair.

One bonus at Northridge that was different from therapy at Topanga was "pet therapy." I didn't know what that was, but it sounded like fun, so I kept an open mind and came to enjoy it. Basically a group of six patients would gather together in a therapy room and a giant volunteer poodle named Nick would join us. Under the supervision of a therapist, we then talked about different topics, while Nick wandered around to each patient to be petted. My speech therapist thought it would be a good idea for me to be a part of such a group setting to practice projecting my voice. At the time, I could only talk very quietly, closer to a whisper.

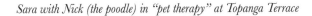

Sara with Nick (the poodle) in "pet therapy" at Topanga Terrace

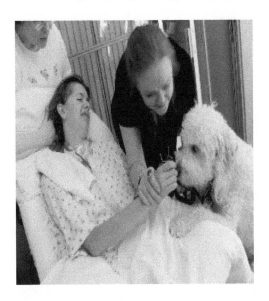

A big part of my therapist's efforts at Northridge was their trying to get me ready to re-enter society again. I was very hesitant to do this because I was embarrassed and ashamed to be in a wheelchair. However, I mustered up the courage and went on a group outing with other patients to the nearby Northridge Mall. My parents drove there too, following the hospital van, in which all the wheelchair patients rode. At the mall, our group first had lunch in the food court. We had to get in line, order the food ourselves and eat at the tables among the general public. Afterwards, my parents and I broke away from the group to do our own browsing. My mom and I first entered Macy's, where I found a diamond and pink sapphire heart necklace in the jewelry section that I really liked. It was close to the holidays so the necklace was on sale. My mom later returned and bought the necklace for me as a Christmas gift from her and my dad. I remember the gift was wrapped in a box under our Christmas tree later that year and it was addressed to "The Survivor."

. That necklace was very special to me because it reminded me of my first trip to the mall in a wheelchair, a big accomplishment. I wanted to return from the mall to the hospital with my parents because it was much more comfortable, but that was against hospital regulations. So I rode back in the van with the other patients. It was quite an ordeal to get everyone loaded into the van because there were several wheelchairs, and they all had to be fastened down. Each wheelchair had a seatbelt at the bottom to fasten the chair to the van floor. Everyone was crammed together in the van. Other than the van ride, the mall trip was a good experience that everyone enjoyed; it felt like a bit of "normalcy" for all of us. We repeated the visit the following week.

I also met someone special at Northridge Hospital. His name was Nick—no, not the poodle, but a young man. Nick was nineteen years old, and he had been involved in a car accident. He was at Northridge learning how to walk again. He didn't have a stroke, so he had totally different physical issues than I did. Every day, he practiced walking with a cane. Nick was an excellent example to me because he was so young and only using a cane temporarily. He even used the cane to walk around at the mall during our outings. I was very resistant to the idea of using a walker or a cane because I thought they were only for old people, and I was in my twenties. Nick helped me to mentally get over that stigma by setting a good example. I hoped that someday I could be a good example to others just as Nick had been to me. I think I may have been one later.

One day I was using a walker, moving down the hallway from the therapy room when I was back in Wisconsin. I approached a little girl, who was maybe five years old at the time. She was in a wheelchair. She pointed at me, which of course was rude, but I was used to getting stares from kids. Then her mom said "Yes, she has a walker just like you, only hers is bigger because she has longer legs." I know it was not for the same problem, but maybe that little girl had noticed that I wasn't very old, and yet I still had to use a walker. Hopefully her mom pointed this out. Maybe she too found some comfort in that, as I did when I saw Nick. I hope so. I also got to know Nick's Mom, Jeanie, and his grandmother, Leila, because they were always with him. I later learned that strong family support was essential to being selected to join Northridge Hospital's rehab program. I certainly had that support from my parents. It's unclear to me why family support was a pre-requisite even though I completely experienced its benefits from my parents. It makes me sympathize with those who don't have this support.

I had "pool therapy" at Northridge, which I didn't have at Topanga because they didn't have a pool. It was quite a process to go to the pool because I needed added assistance to change into my bathing suit and take a shower afterwards. It also took two therapists to escort me into the pool and have sufficient therapy time while in the pool. The pool was kept very warm, so there was no problem adjusting to the temperature. At the time, I couldn't walk, so I would sit on a long wooden board with the therapists. Then we all would be slowly lowered into the water. I really liked being in the water and standing because

I wasn't afraid to fall like I was when I was out of the water. In the water, I could mostly walk alone with little assistance. I took slow and deliberate steps. There was a natural resistance and buoyancy provided by the water. We would practice various things in the pool like walking, sitting in and standing up from a plastic chair submerged in the water, kicking my legs behind me while floating on my stomach, and climbing little steps in the water that divided the pool into levels.

When I returned to Wisconsin to finish my recovery, I was able to continue visiting a therapy pool because my sister Lisa worked at a hospital about ten minutes from my hometown. She was teaching a class at their pool, so I was able to go and do my own therapy with my mom and Lisa nearby. Lisa gave me a square made of pool noodles with handles to put over me to help keep me upright. Using that device was really the only time I could walk by myself without any hands on me to steady me. I really enjoyed pool therapy. Those sessions helped me mentally and physically, as I realized that with time I would hopefully regain my walking ability and walk independently once again.

In Wisconsin, I was also introduced to an aquatic therapy program at the University of Wisconsin-LaCrosse, UWL. The professor, Emmanuel Felix, evaluated me and designed a program for me that I used to practice with the students each week. I really enjoyed my aquatic therapy and working with everyone who was involved in the program. I felt that everyone was doing their best to help get me better. I valued the opportunity of being able to participate in aquatic therapy in addition to all my other therapies. When I carefully climbed down the ladder into the warm therapy water, I was greeted with a pool full of natural buoyancy that surrounded me. Although I was still unbalanced, I felt so much more confident walking in the water than on dry land. While there was always a therapist with me in the water, I didn't really feel like I needed them although I absolutely felt like I needed them out of the water. This balance confidence was something that I desperately wanted out of the water and it was so nice to feel that again during my aquatic therapy.

After five weeks at Northridge, it became a battle with my insurance company to allow me to stay longer. The insurance company evaluated my therapy reports every week to determine if they would pay for an additional week of coverage. By now, I had had more than five months of live-in hospital care. I had virtually exhausted the amount of twenty-four-hour care I could be allotted per my insurance coverage. My parents and I wanted more time at Northridge for the therapy, and even the staff wanted the same for me; I desperately needed it. My therapists, along with Dr. Pigeon, met with an insurance representative and told him how I would greatly benefit by staying there another week. Luckily, my stay was extended that week, and I was very happy with the decision. I was beginning to panic about the thought of going home in a wheelchair. I was planning on walking unassisted after Northridge, but I knew I was still was far away from that happening. I hadn't even considered the possibility of returning home in a wheelchair, but now it was the reality I had to face. So any added time at Northridge was important to me. I could continue to improve a little bit more before I was discharged. Also, I still needed full-time supervision and assistance throughout the day, so my parents would soon have to take over.

Before I left Northridge, I found I was obsessed with time and "How long?" became my favorite question. I would ask everyone, "How long until you think I will walk?" Everyone always answered, "I don't know." "Just give me your best guess,"

I would persist.

No one wanted to give me an answer to avoid being held accountable for my outcome and my timeline. That was very frustrating to me because I just wanted to know the range of what I could expect and when. The therapists who did give me their "best guesses" all said "before Christmas," so I thought it was only going to be another four weeks to regain my balance for walking, and that was a reasonable goal. Looking back, I can say I would have held any doctor or therapist accountable for whatever time guess they gave me. I would have gotten to that time point and told them, "You said I'd be recovered by this point and I'm not, so why not?" Or I would have cried if their guess was too far off. So even though I hated the "I don't know," answer, I also think it was a smart answer and I now understand why I always heard that answer because it was very accurate! Doctors and therapists are amazing, but like anyone else, they don't have all of the answers, and they only can do or say what they know, not what they can predict to make a patient happier.

I can't say how often I heard that "Every stroke is different." And "Let's give it more time." I absolutely hated these responses. I did not meet my Christmas 2009 goal for independent walking to say the least; so after that happened, I stopped giving myself time goals because clearly they were likely to leave me disappointed.

Some of my favorite memories of my time at Northridge were the Sunday drives to the beach. On Sundays, Dr. Pigeon required that I leave the hospital for the afternoon. We went to Zuma beach in Malibu on a couple of those occasions. This was very difficult for me because I had actually been at the beach the day before the stroke happened. On that day, I has been talking to my mom about my constant migraines and watching some dolphins play in the water. On this second visit to the beach, I got out of the car and sat on a blanket on the sand with my parents. It was very emotional because I could remember my last beach visit. Then amazingly, as we sat there, two dolphins swam by very close to shore. It made me happy to see the beach, the ocean and dolphins again and to share this with my parents. On another occasion, we went to Duke's (a restaurant in Malibu) for lunch. Again, it was emotional for me because I had been there in March with my brother, Brian, and his wife, Melanie, when they were visiting me in California.

I was discharged from Northridge on Wednesday, November 18, 2009, as the insurance company no longer deemed me eligible for twenty-four-hour live-in care. They suggested that I live at home and do outpatient care where I would be driven to a hospital a few times a week to do a few hours of therapy and then return home. Such a program meant I would mostly be at home doing my own therapy. I was able to see an outpatient therapist three times after I was discharged. Since I still needed full-time supervision and assistance with washing, dressing, eating, etc., my parents and I thought it would be best for me to return to Wisconsin and live with my mom. My home in Wisconsin was comfortable and familiar to me, and I would be surrounded by extended family and friends. My parents would be much better suited to care for me at their homes in Wisconsin, than they would be in Los Angeles. They also just needed to be home in Wisconsin. They had been living in Los Angeles for nearly six months, and they needed to tend to their own homes and their own lives too. They never mentioned anything about it, but I was very concerned about it and them.

After being discharged, I went back for a handful of days to live in the house Peter and I moved into right before the stroke.

Being in the house again was especially interesting after being away for nearly six months. The week before discharge, per the hospital's suggestion, we visited the house, so it wouldn't be a total shock returning to it when the time came. Entering that house again was extremely emotional. Here I was sitting in a wheelchair, which I could have never imagined would be the case when Peter and I moved in to start our future together. The house was also not handicap accessible, so certain things were a real challenge. Fortunately, the doorways were large enough for a wheelchair to pass through. However, there was no grab bar in the bathroom, and I had become used to one. Nonetheless, I felt a sense of calm and normalcy just being out of the hospital.

The weekend I was discharged also happened to be the weekend that Cary and her son, Kai, visited from Hawaii. It was great to see them again, of course, but I was very humbled by being in a wheelchair. I was certainly better from when Cary saw me in the ICU during my first month. I could not realize that their happiness was seeing me again and how much I had recovered. For them, the wheelchair was not an issue. At least now I could talk quietly with them. Cary even joined me in doing some home exercises. But I also was a long way from where I wanted to be in my recovery journey. Obviously, I thought my condition was going to be much better the next time I saw them, and it was. I just couldn't comprehend it all yet.

Six days later, my parents, Peter, and I boarded a plane for Wisconsin. It was a Tuesday, November 24, and just a couple days before Thanksgiving.

CHAPTER 15

"When You Say Wis-Con-Sin…"

WAS EXCITED to return to Wisconsin for several reasons. I guess there's just something about "going home" that is just so comfortable and familiar. I grew up in Wisconsin, I love Wisconsin, and despite the apprehension I was feeling for the reason why I was returning home, it was still home for me and I loved it. Also, most importantly for me, I was able to "return" my parents to Wisconsin. They had been in California tending to me for nearly six months, and I felt very guilty about it. In addition, I certainly did not want them to spend the coming holidays away from family. I was also very excited to return to Wisconsin and be closer to family and friends and completely away from any hospital environment. Finally, we all thought that living in a home setting would do me a lot of good.

I grew up in Western Wisconsin, in Westby. The next big city near Westby is LaCrosse, which borders Minnesota with the Mississippi river splitting the two states. I'd like to describe the town where I grew up. It's Westby, Wisconsin. I am definitely a small-town girl. Westby has a little over 2,000 people. We only have two stoplights in the whole county, neither of which is in Westby. Stoplights are not to be confused with stop signs, of which we do have plenty. Westby is of Norwegian heritage, and our little stores certainly represent that history. For example, we have the Uff-da Mart and Dregne's Scandinavian Gifts, Nordic Lanes and Borgen's Cafe.

Our taxi picked us up at 5 a.m. We had a ton of luggage plus the wheelchair and the walker. We left Los Angeles at 8 a.m. on a beautiful November morning heading to Wisconsin. I was nervous about my future. I had been indefinitely ripped away from my life and now found myself in a wheelchair and totally dependent on everyone. To say the least, I was terrified about returning to Wisconsin in a wheelchair because I grew up there, and everyone knew me.

After the first leg of our trip and a long trek through the Minneapolis airport, we found the gate that said "LaCrosse," our final destination. We were almost home. When the plane finally touched down there, it was a wonderful feeling, especially for my parents who had spent so much time with me in California. I was very apprehensive about coming home in a wheelchair and seeing my family and friends that way. However, everyone treated me the same, so I had nothing to worry about. We had to wait for everyone to get off the plane of course, so my wheelchair could be brought up from the luggage area of the plane. Finally, we were able to disembark. As my mom wheeled me down the ramp and through the gate I saw my family waiting for me. We were greeted by my sister, Lisa, her three kids Tyler, Tanner, Isabella, my Grandma Sieber (my mom's mom), my aunt Sandy, my mom's friend, Dwain, and our family friend, Beth. I remember Mom saying to me "Lisa brought the kids!" We weren't sure if that was going to happen, as the airport is about fifty minutes from home, the kids were still in school, and it would be a late night for them.

It was a very emotional return. We took a lot of time for hugs and tears. Our return was a huge milestone—I had defied all the odds. I had finally come home. After we got our luggage, we met my brother, Brian, a postal carrier at the time, was working near the airport. I hadn't seen Brian for several months. We were really happy to be home and with family again. We had arrived in Wisconsin just a couple of days before Thanksgiving. On this Thanksgiving, I celebrated at home with my family. It was a special celebration because these years there were many special reasons to give thanks. Usually, I wouldn't have returned to Wisconsin for Thanksgiving. I would have waited until mid-December when the teaching semester was over. I couldn't even remember the last Thanksgiving I spent in Wisconsin because I had lived for the last five years in either California or Hawaii.

My recovery was clearly dependent on three things: patience, positivity, and persistence. I felt I definitely had all three. I had to be really patient and then do hours of daily therapy for years to even vaguely near my ambitious goal of normalcy, which most doctors and therapists told me was unachievable. Luckily, I've always been a very positive person, as are my parents, so I knew I had that part on my side. Finally, I was very persistent. I never gave up despite how long I had to wait or how frustrated I got sometimes. I can attribute my recovery to more, but these three qualities were my constants, my personal philosophy and my mantra.

One thing I was often told by doctors and therapists was that age was on my side. I was happy to hear this detail, but I wanted my youth to make my recovery faster. It didn't. There were people older than I who recovered from their strokes faster, and I was less than half their age! I kept wondering when my recovery would speed up. However, I focused instead on the knowledge that it was my age that was allowing me to regain so much post-stroke. Also, my recovery struggle was a demonstration of just how devastating my stroke actually was. It's hard for me to comprehend how close I was to death. Finally, as frustrating as it is, stroke is a brain injury. I also knew that the brain is amazing. It just heals very slowly, but IT CAN HEAL!

Arriving in Wisconsin, I knew I would be there for a while, so it was important to find a good home therapy routine. I wanted to get out of that wheelchair as soon as possible. However, I could not start scheduled therapy at the hospital until January 1, 2010, because of the insurance. The insurance I had in California was not accepted in Wisconsin, so USC, my former employer, let me change to another insurance that was accepted in Wisconsin. It just wouldn't become effective until January 1, 2010. So I had to create my own home program for December.

That home program consisted of floor exercises (crunches, leg lifts, arm raises, etc.) and walking back and forth across the kitchen, with my parents holding my hands. I was scared to walk because I was always scared of falling and getting badly hurt. My parents were also highly concerned that if I fell, I could break something and have a major setback. I felt very off balance as well. So I was resistant to walking when we first arrived home. My parents almost had to force me to walk. But I did.

Many therapists tried to encourage me to use special adaptations to make my life easier. However, I was too stubborn to accept most of their suggestions. Mom had a grab bar installed in the bathroom as well as a portable shower attachment, and she placed a lawn chair in the shower, so I could sit down when I showered. She did not want a ramp installed outside our house for the wheelchair, because I was really resistant to anything seen as "not normal" or stroke related. Thus, we had larger stairs made with a railing installed to go into the house. Fortunately, our home is one story, so I didn't have to worry about any other stairs. I was disabled, of course, but only temporarily in all our eyes, so I didn't want anything that catered to my disability. I refused raised toilet seats (makes the toilet seat higher when sitting), and refused food plates with ridges to push the food against, bigger kitchen utensils, a clip-on microphone to project my quiet voice, and a computer program with voice recognition to help me type. I didn't want to rely on any of them. Honestly, I know now they would have made life much easier for me then, but I was just too stubborn to accept them. Instead, I wanted to do things normally even if doing so took me longer. Fortunately for me, my parents were willing to keep everything as normal as possible in the face of everything about me being abnormal. They had infinite patience and I know now that their determination and faith in me were the keys to my recovery.

CHAPTER 16

Let's Stretch!

FINALLY BEGAN the scheduled hospital therapy again at Gundersen Lutheran Hospital in LaCrosse, Wisconsin. I knew that therapy would be necessary for a long time. Fortunately, I really liked my therapists. I knew then, and I still believe that it is so important to like your therapists. It makes a world of difference mentally, and mental positivity helps you physically. I thought my therapists were extremely nice, and I could tell they liked me too. It was really good to know they were all on my team, and they all shared the same goal as me—full recovery.

In addition to the hospital therapy, my vigorous home workout program now seemed to get longer and more intense, as I added the exercises I did in therapy. I want to give you an example of my program during a small period of my life. However, it should be noted that this particular schedule did NOT last forever, and my home exercise routine varied greatly, depending on what I wanted to focus on at home. The routine I'm about to describe probably lasted a few weeks, and then I would switch it up further. Don't expect another stroke patient to match my exact routine because I created this routine based on my therapy experience and my ability at this time. I think it's best that everyone has a bit of autonomy in creating their own routine in order to maintain motivation.

First, I would start with an hour routine right after waking up in bed because while lying down, I was in a good position to do many exercises. At first, my workout in bed consisted of only leg lifts because all my therapists said my left hip was weak and needed more attention. Leg lifts were one exercise that made my hip hurt, so I thought it must be really effective, which is what Dad always said. Soon, I added many more exercises to my bed routine, so a session that started as ten minutes quickly turned into over an hour of exercise, all done right after waking up! I remember thinking it was going to be a good day when I finally could wake up and didn't immediately have to begin my day by exercising in bed.

My normal routine began with 60 regular crunches, holding each for 10 seconds, 100 bicycle crunches holding each for two seconds, and 60 bridges holding each for 10 seconds. A bridge is when you lie on your back but your legs are bent while keeping your feet on the floor. Next you push into your heels, flex your glutes together and lift your pelvis off the floor. Then, I did 120 triceps lifts with a one pound weighted ball, very slow and con-trolled, and 60 wrist bends with the same weighted one pound ball, using both hands. I did 60 left leg lifts holding each for 10 seconds. Then I would use a therapy clothespin with much more resistance than a regular clothespin, with hands, thumb and each finger 25 times for a total of 100. I then squeezed my hand using a hand-gripper 100 times. I also usually did the gripper and the clothespin at the same time, one in each hand to save time. This did not make it physically more difficult, it was just more difficult to concentrate.

Next, Dad would help me get up from bed and walk around inside the house for about thirty minutes. He would hold a gait belt around my waist while I used a walker or a cane. The treadmill work followed for about thirty minutes. Then, I would have breakfast. I always tried to eat using a fork with my left (affected) hand. That was very hard, and I quickly abandoned it because of the difficulty. After breakfast, I would do an eye-tracking program on the computer for my misaligned eyes for around fifteen minutes. Whenever my eyes saw certain cues on the screen, I would use my left hand to hit the space bar. Then, I would type with both hands for fifteen minutes. That was my hardest and least favorite therapy because of my slow left hand.

I also practiced handwriting because the coordination center in my brain had been severely affected by the stroke, making my handwriting sloppier. I had a handwriting notebook, and I would date every day, so I could track my progress. I basically had to relearn how to write again. Right after the stroke, I could only make very basic marks on the paper, and everything was ineligible at first. For handwriting practice, I would print the alphabet three times, the numbers 1 through 20 and my name three times. Eventually, I practiced writing in cursive (which was more difficult) the full names of my immediate family members. Once that task was completed, I would go to the bathroom and brush my teeth using my left hand to start, which was also very hard! I always used my right hand to finish that task to ensure I did a good job. However, I also quickly abandoned this task due to its difficulty.

After breakfast I would do balancing and muscle building exercises at "the bar." My parents had bought a chin-up bar, which they installed at hip-level across a doorway. I could hold on to it. I would do a routine of balance exercises using the bar for support. I would start with marching in place sixty times, which was good practice at shifting my weight. Many people who have balance issues from a stroke have a hard time with weight shifting, so this exercise was an important one for me to do. My dad would get on the other side of the bar and wrap a therapy rubber band around each thigh and I would bend my knee, and then straighten it. Next came fifty squats and thirty calf and toe raises. Then I did forty kick outs and backs with each leg, followed by twenty lunges with each leg, while holding the bar and my dad's hand to steady myself. After all of this I would take a break for lunch. It probably took three or four hours to get to this point in my day. After lunch, I would do thirty more minutes of walking, and ten more minutes on a treadmill if I could talk my dad into it, which was rare.

My parents and my therapists had an interesting point of view in their interactions with me. Instead of talking me into exercise, they were often talking me out of exercise. Even Kathy, my physical therapist at the time, said I was the hardest working patient she had ever seen in her career. I thought their views were great to know. My parents would often say, "Sara, you're done. No more exercise today. Tomorrow's another day." I would say, "Don't punish me by taking away my exercise!" Sometimes I was sad when they had to cut me off, but other times I was happy because I was tired. When I was on the treadmill, I would often plead with them to make it go faster or let me walk longer. However, it was tiring for them too because they needed to stand by the machine and hold on to my gait belt to steady me against any possible fall. Sometimes my parents would stop the therapy because they were tired, not me. I was never the one to say I was too tired to do something. Actually, once I did say I was tired, and they made me stop, so I quickly learned never to say this word to them. I think my dedicated mindset had a lot to do with the exercise routine I was already used to doing before I had the stroke.

I had especially embraced cardio, so it was easier for me to want to do similar cardio exercises after the stroke. In contrast, I had hated strength training before, so now I had to talk myself into doing a regular routine of strengthening moves during my recovery. I felt that my daily exercise routine for recovery was quite intensive, and it was. But that 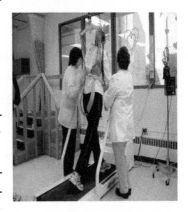 was what I wanted to do to get better. It's hard to imagine all of the ways a stroke affects your body.

My sister Lisa works at Vernon Memorial Hospital, which was also where I visited a gym. One day when I was there, she was giving heel bone density scans, so she gave me one. Despite all the exercise I was doing at home and at therapy, my results were still not that great. This was because regardless of my commitment to doing all my therapy, due to my poor balance, I simply was not on my feet as much as a "normal" person my age would be every day. We chose a more involved bone density scan and kept a close eye on it, and everything ended up being okay. I do think it's important for any stroke patient to be conscious of this issue, to be fully aware of how important weight-bearing exercises are for bone health, and to try to add more of this weight bearing efforts into your day, even if it's just standing with a walker.

I did take breaks from therapy sometimes. Dad tried to take me out for a drive often to get me out of the house and away from therapy for a while. Westby is surrounded by beautiful scenery, so we often took the back roads on our drives to view the country-side. Many Amish live in the area and it's fun to see them in their horse-drawn carriages. They are always so friendly and wave as they go by. I didn't want to go to retail stores of course because I was so embarrassed about my eye misalignment and my bad balance. I knew there was a good chance I would see someone I knew in a store, and I really didn't want that to happen because of my insecurity. I thoroughly enjoyed these drives together with my dad. They were my treasured, wonderful "escape" from therapy.

I struggled a great deal to see more progress, and I found myself living my own "comeback" story. My goal was to be back exactly to how I was before the stroke, just like Jen, the girl I described here who also had a stroke, but recovered so well. I realize that it sounds like I had an unrealistic or lofty goal, but that's what it was. I decided to fight for that goal as best I could, and I listened to all the therapists who said they had seen people in my shoes before, or similar shoes. I felt like such a disappointment to my parents, but whenever I brought that feeling up, they would tell me just the opposite. They would tell me they were so very proud of me. Dad would often ask, "Does it seem easier?" I would always say, "No." He would then say, "It must!"

I honestly couldn't see my own progress, so I just blindly trusted my parents and therapists who insisted that they did. Even my occupational therapist in LaCrosse, Tami, couldn't believe that I couldn't see any difference after several months because she thought it was so obvious. There's one thing that I now really feel bad about saying: When I was at Topanga Terrace was going to move to Northridge Hospital, Dr. Pigeon asked me, "Aren't you happy you stayed at Topanga longer and you made more progress?"

"No." I replied.

I honestly couldn't see any progress, but I did have awesome therapists at Topanga. My telling Dr. Pigeon that I didn't see any progress was me saying I couldn't speak highly of their work. I regretted saying it, and should have complimented their work because they all deserved that praise. In retrospect, I now realize that some of my bad behavior was the result of the effects of the stroke on my brain. Observing my progress was always very subjective for me, so I was happy when the therapists used objective tests to measure my progress by scoring and timing me in various activities. I could clearly see progress when I saw those objective tests.

Because of this blindness to my progress, Kathy, my physical therapist in Wisconsin, told me that I had "selective memory." She would ask, "Don't you remember your first day here? You were using the walker, and it was all over the place." "No." I would respond. I remembered using the walker, but not when I didn't have any control of the walker.

Dad would also ask me when we were practicing our bar exercises, "Do you remember not being able to do any lunges?"

"No," I would respond. Similarly, I never remembered not being able to do lunges. I sometimes wished I could remember the bad parts because that would have helped me see that all of my hard work was paying off. But then I would reconsider and realize I was very happy I didn't remember some of those bad parts because those are not memories I want. However, I honestly couldn't see my own progress. Kathy said I should celebrate even small victories because my goal of achieving perfection was either unattainable or very far away. Still, my progress was so slow that I couldn't even celebrate small victories because I couldn't identify them. It was thus easier to identify that I was moving forward based on the objective tests we did in therapy. It was only through seeing actual scores or times that I could see I was making actual real progress.

I started to have a recurring dream. While the situations varied in the dream, one detail remained the same. I couldn't open my eyes. Later, I would physically try to open my eyes in the dream, but when I did, I was blind. This dream occurred often over several months, and it was very frustrating. I searched on the Internet for what it meant and found that it likely meant that I couldn't see something in my life. I honestly didn't know what that could be. Then, one night I was telling my mom about the dream, and I realized what it was. "Of course! I can't see my progress!" It seemed obvious then. I started to respond "yes" or "slowly, but surely" when people asked if I was improving. The dreams went away. I had wanted to see my progress so badly prior to that dream but I just couldn't. I thought it was interesting that my subconscious forced me to see what was going on. I was making strides towards real progress every day.

A large part of seeing my progress was paying attention to my objective therapy scores. In occupational therapy, OT, they would do a grip test where I would squeeze a gripper to determine my hand strength. They would do the same with a pinch test. Then, I would be timed while putting small pegs into the holes of a board, then taking them out as quickly as I could. This was a test to measure my coordination skill. I would also practice typing with both hands, and that action was also timed. These tests were performed each month, and my scores were documented, so each month I could actually "see" my progress. Even though I struggled to see my progress daily, I could still see my scores monthly, and that was very helpful to let me now identify the progress I was making.

It is always hard to maintain motivation doing anything when you can't see clear results. So I trusted my parents and therapists, and I often thought of my friend Jen, who had recovered so well from her stroke. They all kept me going and encouraging my doing the monotonous exercises. Sometimes my therapy times would be slower than the day, week, or month earlier. That was upsetting, but I would always try to remember that variations in progress were to be expected, so all I could do was keep trying. My physical therapist in LaCrosse thought my goal was perfection, which it was, but that made it even harder to see my actual progress.

Similar to occupational therapy, in physical therapy we also did an objective test. It was called the Berg Balance Scale, another objective test that helped me see my progress. In this test, I would do different balance tests to determine how much of a risk I was at for falling. In these tests I would stand with my eyes closed, stand and look over my shoulders, stand on one leg without holding on to anything (which was very hard), and other tests. I was very happy when I finally graduated into a low fall risk category, although I disagreed that I was a low fall risk. I felt that I really should still be considered a high risk due to my lack of balance. There were some things in physical therapy, however, where I knew I had made big improvements, like having the therapists remove the harness that held me upright while I would walk on the treadmill or graduating from the walker to the quad cane, and then from the quad cane to the single-point cane, and then finally from the single-point cane to no device at all. Even though I couldn't see my progress from day to day, I could still see these jumps in my abilities.

I am absolutely a positive testament to stroke progress continuing well after a year. With strokes, there is no cutoff date for progress. Every stroke and its subsequent recovery period will vary per individual. I can say now that my stroke progress has never stopped, and it took me several years after my stroke to become independent again. That may seem disheartening to some because even at my young age, it took so long, but it did happen! My stroke was incredibly massive, and it nearly killed me! I think it is hopeful to many others to know my story and realize that hard work and determination can get you there.

I also heard that after a year you cannot expect too much in terms of results. I remember thinking I sure hope that's untrue! Kathy, my physical therapist at the time, told me to never believe that progress stops after a year. Even after a year, I was still largely dependent. I was practicing walking by myself, but it was very slow and deliberate. In fact it wasn't really "by myself" since someone was always behind me holding on to the gait belt around my waist. I mean I had no assistive device. I once asked Kathy, my PT, "Have I plateaued?" She and my dad laughed. Dad kept laughing about my question even after therapy that day because he thought it was totally ridiculous. I was serious because I was blind to my progress then, but I was very happy that they had found my question so comical.

My parents and I struggled with how to let go of me while walking. Obviously the safest choices would have been to have me stay in a wheelchair or have someone with me at all times for the rest of my life. That wasn't feasible, so we had to find a way for them to trust me and hope I wouldn't fall. Mom said she was told to expect a fall. She hoped that would not happen if someone was with me all the time. I did fall a few times, but luckily I never was seriously hurt. She always worried that if I did get hurt in a fall, it might be a disaster. For example, if I got a sprain or broke an ankle, that kind of injury would have set me back several weeks or even months. I hated it when I did fall because my parents blamed themselves, even though it was always only my fault. Even my physical therapist, Kathy, agreed. She said if I ever fell, it was always my fault. However, my falling made it much harder to try again and also gain my parents' trust again. Falling was hard on me too because it increased my fear of falling again. I learned that the balance center in my brain was very hard to retrain, but very slowly and surely, it was learning the lessons I was teaching it.

Dad said when we first came back from California I would walk a lap (about twenty steps) with the walker. He said I would have fallen every time, had he not been with me. With time, we got to a point where he wouldn't have to catch me at all even when not using any device! I remember being very resistant to the walker and canes because I thought they were only for old people, and I was in my twenties, but then once again, I thought of Nick from Northridge who was only nineteen and had to use a cane. I definitely saw his cane as temporary, and a means for him to get back to walking independently. I decided that his path would be my path too towards getting the long-term improvement I wanted.

I must admit that Dad was much braver than Mom and more ready to let me move independently. Mom was too scared that I would fall and get hurt, setting my recovery back. Dad was scared too, but he knew I had to go it alone sometime, so he was more willing to take that risk than Mom was, to let me try to improve my balance by myself.

Ultimately, Wisconsin helped me rehabilitate myself. I spent years doing extensive therapy to physically become more independent. I also spent years immersed in such a loving environment back home in humble Wisconsin and realized that this is where I truly belong and desire to be. I had to focus on the many physical deficits I did have. However, equally important were all other challenges I had faced, as you'll learn in the next chapter of my story.

CHAPTER 17

"...You've Said It All"

FTER ESTABLISHING MY therapy program in Wisconsin, I learned there were many other aspects of my stroke recovery that I still had to deal with and overcome. Many of these issues were social or emotional aspects I had to handle personally in order to fully rehabilitate. I never would have thought twice about any of these issues pre-stroke because I never struggled with them. However, after my stroke, I was presented with numerous emotional challenges I also had to overcome.

I struggled with appropriateness at times. To be more specific, I would often think, what is the most inappropriate thing I could say or do right now? I never acted on this thought. However, when I believed I was stuck in a nightmare, I tried to act inappropriately to try to end the dream. For example, I would say something completely untrue or deliberately hurtful to try to end that dream. Fortunately, I finally recognized that these impulses of inappropriateness were solely caused by the stroke. Therefore, I would think, I'm not going to say or do anything inappropriate because that would be the stroke getting the best of me. I know this reason sounds very simple, but it did help me immensely because I was so determined to beat the stroke in the end. As time went on, I could tell that my inappropriate urges were lessening their grip on me. I believed I should be excused from my stroke rehab behavior, but now I think this should have been applied a little more generally. I thought I should be excused for the rest of my life from anything inappropriate because I had brain damage. Of course, this is just my opinion, and now I say it a bit tongue in cheek.

Anonymity was very important to me. In fact, my favorite part about moving to Northridge Hospital from Topanga Terrace was anonymity. I loved that no one knew me. Because Topanga Terrace is a nursing home, and I was only twenty-seven, I stood out, and everyone knew me and my story. At Northridge Hospital, there was a mix of ages, so I could blend in better. In Westby, Dad and I were walking at the high-school track one day when a man, who I didn't know, asked Dad right in front of me, "What's wrong with your daughter?" I thought the question was incredibly rude. Further, one time my mom and brother were helping me walk from church when another man asked my brother, "What's wrong with her?" The worst time, however, was when I was walking to therapy at UWL, and an older woman, who was using a cane passed me, and right afterwards she told someone next to her, well within earshot of me, "It's always nice to see someone worse off than yourself." It really hurt my feelings to hear this. Not only was this rude, but I completely disagreed! I don't think it's "nice" to see someone else worse off than you are.

On the other hand, many other people noticed me and commended me. The vast majority of comments to me were positive compliments. However, early on in my recovery, I used to cry when anyone would compliment me because I was embarrassed to be pointed out even if it was in a positive way. Further into my rehab, I started to get a little sassier when people asked me unintentionally rude questions like, "Were you in a car accident?" I would respond with something like, "It's not your concern. I know you don't mean anything by it, but that's a rude question, and you shouldn't ask that of anyone." I felt like I needed to protect other individuals from being asked these same questions from nosy individuals. It is never polite to ask or comment on another's hardships, no matter how you choose to phrase that comment.

As time passed, I became more and more proud of what I was doing and finally could graciously accept compliments with a simple, "Thank you." Being pointed out made me feel different initially. It really didn't matter to me who the person was—a therapist, doctor or even another disabled individual. I never felt it was appropriate to point me out, and again, it is never polite to ask what happened to someone. I remembered this later on when I would see someone disabled and wanted to inquire as to what happened but I would remember how I felt and how no one should ask this. Sometimes, if I was walking well, Dad would say, "It looks like you just have a bad ankle now." I always liked when he said it because my goal was to be completely "normal" again.

Another common comment made to me was people telling me about other people's strokes. I fully realize that these people were only trying to be helpful and I would have appreciated these stories more had they been good examples of how the stroke patient completely rebounded from a stroke. However, whenever I asked, "How are they today?" I almost always heard, "They still have deficits." Now why would anyone retell that kind of story to me? So I could interpret that despite my hard work I'd still have deficits? When people would say, "After twenty years, he or she's still improving," I was happy to hear that progress was still occurring. But I also wanted to be done with my own stroke rehab in less than twenty years. Then, I recognized the truth. I would be dealing with my stroke deficits my whole life, so I started to focus on the thought that it was possible to get to ninety percent recovery now, then finish the remaining ten percent during the rest of my life. I was at peace with that idea, even if I had just invented it.

I love language, so let's focus on it briefly here. There were certain words I didn't like used around me at the beginning of my recovery. The first word was "progress." I thought it was overused and inaccurate when talking about me. I also hated the word "relearn" because I didn't think I was relearning anything. My brain fortunately still knew how to do everything because the stroke had not damaged that part of my brain. My parents said that if I discarded one word, I had to provide a suitable alternative, so for "relearn" I decided "retrain" was more accurate. I didn't mind "good" or "bad" instead of "unaffected" and "affected," respectively, although some therapists are often told not to say "good" or "bad" when referring to the sides of the body after a stroke. I remember one time I was doing something to practice with my hands, and my mom saw me "cheating" by using my right hand and not doing the complete movement with both hands.

She told me, "Sara, you're only cheating yourself."

I thought the comment was unfair, as I was just trying to get through the exercise. Then I realized I was not only cheating myself; I was also cheating my parents, my family and my friends who were all cheering long and hard for me. I tried to remember this as an exercise motivator since I despised the monotonous hand exercises and never wanted to do them.

Another language clarification I would make here is substituting compensate for cheat. Therapists often said I was cheating on an exercise by favoring my right (stronger) side. I would then say, "No, I'm just compensating." I was never intentionally trying to cheat. I was just trying to complete the exercise, and my body was trying to do it as well by relying more on my stronger side to do so.

Many people told me I was an "inspiration." While this is a wonderful word, I thought it was used very loosely to describe me. I didn't ever argue with anyone about it because I thought if I made someone's day easier or made someone not take something they could already do for granted, then it was great.

Olympic athletes are inspirations. My friend Windi is an inspiration because she has maintained such a positive attitude despite her permanent disability. My friend Emmanuel is an inspiration for his unwavering commitment to better himself and live his life to the fullest. I didn't feel like I was an inspiration. However, it isn't a bad thing to be considered an inspiration. I always enjoyed being considered one.

During my daily rehab, I always repeated different proverbs over and over again in my head because I felt they were appropriate. Such examples are "patience is a virtue" because I had to be so incredibly patient throughout my recovery efforts. "Whatever doesn't kill you only makes you stronger" for obvious reasons, "Practice makes perfect" and of course, "Try, try again." The last two I would tell myself especially when I stumbled while walking. Every day, I felt like I had to brush myself off and try again. I had always prided myself before the stroke for being a strong, capable, and independent person. I didn't want to have to depend on anyone or to be anyone's burden. After the stroke, I was a burden to many because I needed help with nearly everything, so I had to accept that I was going to be a burden for a while. But I never lost the hope that eventually I wouldn't be a burden to anyone in the future.

One issue I suffered from after the stroke that was surprising to me and everyone around me was being diagnosed with depression. It was surprising because I have always been a positive person and anyone who knows me would describe me as always positive and happy. An anti-depressant seemed like the last thing I would ever need. However, my doctors felt I needed one for several months post-stroke. It was because initially, I cried so much it would sometimes interrupt my therapy. I could tell the difference when I was taking the medicine and when I was not. I would never have described myself as an "emotional" individual before the stroke. However, after the stroke, I noticed a shift to where I felt more emotional sometimes.

With a cerebellar stroke of the type I had suffered, I learned that control of my body was a big deficit of mine, even the control of my emotions. Not every tear was one of sadness either. I noticed myself wiping away tears sometimes just watching videos of my nieces and nephews. I actually felt a little ashamed to be on an anti-depressant. However, I had to remind myself it wasn't permanent, and I had been through an awful lot! When

I was trying to get off the medication I did so slowly! That meant getting a pill cutter and cutting the medication in half, so it wouldn't reduce too quickly. When I had tried to reduce it too quickly, I cried for no reason. One time I even tried to stop entirely, and even though it was done slowly, it was premature and it just interrupted my therapy again. So I restarted the medicine for a while before finally stopping again. The doctor allowed me to reduce the dose by half every six weeks when I was stopping the medication.

However, as I mentioned earlier here, instead of depression, I was most likely suffering from pseudobulbur affect (PBA). I previously described how PBA is a neurological condition that explains bouts of inappropriate crying. This made more sense to me because although I had every reason to be depressed, I really didn't feel like I was. Even years into my recovery, I would have naturally preferred to be a lot further along than I was, but I was still quite happy overall. Therefore I have never really believed the "depression" diagnosis.

In addition to crying more than usual, I also apologized more than usual. Many times, I apologized three times in a row. "Sorry, sorry, sorry." Usually, I apologized for my bad balance. That was because whoever was with me, usually my parents or a therapist, would have to catch me if I fell or lost my balance. I felt I was a burden because of this problem, so I was always apologizing. Even when I was in therapy, and we were trying to challenge my balance, I would still apologize when I lost my balance. I remember, one time at therapy, I was walking, and I stumbled a bit. The therapist had to rebalance me, so I apologized. She sarcastically said, "Yes Sara, you should be sorry." I thought her retort was funny because I knew I was apologizing too much, and yet I still felt I should. It was more like a reflex for me—stumble, and then apologize. A yoga instructor of mine, Carol Anne Kemen, was the only person who ever called me out on it. When we were doing yoga together one day, she said, "Why did you apologize just now?" She didn't see any reason for it. I explained that I felt I was too slow moving on to the next exercise. I knew there really was no need, but that's a good example of how I'd often apologize for unnecessary things.

I was also jealous of little kids' abilities because they were so small and they could do so much more than I could. I never would have traded places with anyone or wished my condition on anyone, but many times I did wish my abilities were further along. I would watch my niece and nephews, Tyler (nine), Tanner (six), and Isabella (three) freely run and see how easy it was for them, while there I was practicing little steps, hoping it might become automatic and easier for me to just walk again. Later, my brother, Brian, and his wife, Melanie, had three daughters, Arianna, Madison, and Elise, and I watched as they learned to walk sooner than me. I was of course very proud of them, but it was humbling at the same time.

I remember the kids were over at my mom's house one night, and my mom brought out a bunch of old children's toys from when I was little. I needed practice with my left arm and children's toys make great tools. Isabella was taking some rings off a stand using both her arms, when I thought, *I hope I get to that point one day.* I've learned that kids are great because they don't care about physical differences. Tyler, Tanner, and Isabella still treated me like the same aunt I was before the stroke and that was a great feeling for me to have.

As I previously mentioned, I was terribly insecure after the stroke. Initially, it was mostly because of my eyes. My third and fifth cranial nerves were severely affected by the stroke. As a result, my left eye looked straight on, but my right eye was stuck in the outer corner of my eye. Because of this issue, I was very embarrassed, and it was a large part of why I was resistant to visitors for so long. I realize now that this was a vanity issue, but it was very embarrassing for me! I now realize that my friends and family were just happy that I was alive. How I looked was completely unimportant to them. Appearances are superficial and there was so much love around me and everyone celebrated my progress. I realized that everyone truly loved the "inside of Sara," which was great to feel.

When we consulted doctors in California on this issue after the stroke, they always told me, "We don't know how much the eyes will correct themselves naturally, so let's wait until a year after the stroke before we make any decisions on surgery." This kind of response was typical and highly frustrating for me because "time" was out of my control and time seemed to be the only answer I was given. It was also frustrating for me because several therapists seemed to think that this misalignment of my eyes also negatively affected my walking balance, which I was trying so hard at the time to correct.

So I did what I could to naturally encourage my eyes to improve. My therapist encouraged me to use an eye tracking program on my computer, which I used for nearly seven months. This program was about fifteen minutes long, and you had to hit the space bar when you saw the object pass by on the screen. It was very boring, but I did it anyway. I also wore an eye patch over one eye (often for two hours per day) to try to strengthen my right eye and I practiced other-eye tracking exercises every day to try to stretch the eye muscle. Despite all of these efforts, however, I saw no difference in my eye alignment. We were all tired of waiting to see the needed improvement with my eye alignment and overall vision, especially me.

Post-stroke, I noticed it was more difficult to see, especially to see small lettering clearly. I thought my vision was a little better in my right eye, but that eye was stuck in the corner, so I had to tilt my head a lot and try to look through my right eye more of the time. This head tilting was because I could move my neck better than I could move my eye muscles.

We went to see an eye doctor in January 2010, and she gave me a prescription for glasses. It was a much smaller prescription than I had required pre-PRK. She attributed my vision loss to the stroke, since my third cranial nerve was paralyzed and my eye alignment was obviously affected and also because I had been seeing fine without a prescription before the stroke and after PRK. The glasses did help me stop tilting my head because I no longer thought I had to tilt it in order to see well. I had no idea how much damage the stroke had done to my eyes.

After fourteen months, we decided to explore a possible surgical procedure. When my mom went to see her ophthalmologist in the spring, she asked him, "If one of your family members had a problem with an eye, who would you, see?" He gave her the name of a doctor at the Mayo Clinic in Rochester, Minnesota, about two hours' driving distance from where we lived. I was very excited because Mayo has such a strong reputation. And I was so sick of living with my eyes looking so weird. When we contacted the neuro-opthomologist, we provided a copy of my medical records. And Mom also wrote a description of what had happened to me.

Once we were "pre-approved," we arranged the visits to see a neuro-opthomologist. I had seen two ophthalmologists previously, and both had said, "We need to wait at least a year to see how much natural return we can get with the eye."

I hated this response. To me it sounded like "I have no idea; let's wait at least a year until you find someone who knows what they're talking about." We went to an appointment and after a long exam, the doctor leaned back in his chair and said, "I'm not your guy for this surgery but I can introduce you to your guy." He led us to a different office and introduced us to Dr. Brodsky.

Dr. Brodsky and his assistant took several measurements. He works a lot with children and small babies so he had a bouncing dragon on his light to distract them from the exam. After this exam, he stood back and said, "I can help you." My parents and I were so happy to hear this from a doctor. I remember my heart soaring when I heard those words. I was elated. I felt it would improve not only my physical appearance, but also remove many of my emotional issues because I was so embarrassed about my eyes. In addition, it could improve my eye alignment and therefore, hopefully my balance and coordination as well.

Overall, I was very happy and excited about the surgery and only slightly hesitant about the small, but possible, risk of loss of vision. For me, the potential benefits far outweighed the risks. The doctor told me that double vision would be very likely because my eyes had been misaligned for so long that my brain had probably adjusted to it, so it could take a while for the eyes to readjust in the months after surgery. My eyes would also be very red for a couple of weeks. They also said it would be very possible to need a second surgery, but they would have to wait at least two months post-surgery to determine that. Regardless of the precautions, I was very excited. We scheduled a surgery the same day.

My left eye had had alignment issues my whole life. At age two, I was diagnosed has having a wandering eye, as opposed to a lazy eye. When I was little, they didn't want to do anything to correct it because the doctor at the time said I would want to be able to control it as I grew older. I did just that, but if I got tired, it was very difficult for me to control it. In that instance, my left eye would "wander" to the outer corner of my eye while my right eye remained straight.

After the stroke, the situation changed. My left eye was frozen straight, but my right eye didn't "wander," it was simply stuck in the right corner of my eye. I had no control over this situation, even after months of eye exercises. I didn't experience double vision after my eye surgery and the doctor said the most likely reason for this was my previous experience dealing with an eye misalignment. My brain was already able to recognize and pro-cess a similar misalignment, so my past history actually ended up being a blessing in disguise to prevent double vision after my post-stroke eye surgery.

The surgery date arrived, and we traveled to the Mayo Clinic in Rochester, Minnesota. The Mayo Clinic is arguably the best clinic worldwide for healthcare, and that knowledge comforted us all. People travel from all over the world to be treated there. We were happy that we lived only a couple of hours away. When we got to Mayo, we could sense its size and value, starting with its impressive waiting room. Unfortunately, I had become a very good judge of hospitals. When you enter the lobby at Mayo, it is huge, open, and entirely marbled. It feels expensive. There are two buildings that are connected, and both are nineteen stories: the Mayo building and the Gonda building. My eye surgery was actually performed at St. Mary's Hospital, at a different location in the same city. When we arrived for the surgery and after we checked in, we were given a hospital bed and a room, similar to what I had received at Northridge Hospital and Topanga Terrace. We were again reminded how nice it was not to be living in that former setting. My doctor, Dr. Brodsky, would be performing the surgery, and he visited me at my bedside. We were surprised and pleased to see him before the surgery. I was a little apprehensive, but mostly, I was excited to be having surgery on my eyes.

I asked Mom, "Do you have any bad feelings?" I was pretty sure she would have had bad feelings if something bad were going to happen to me.

"No, I think you'll be fine," she replied and smiled.

Had she said "I feel nervous and I think we should leave," I would have listened. I know that may sound silly, but I trust my mother's intuition completely.

My eye surgery was called "strabismus" surgery. It was meant to improve the alignment of my eyes, which was so affected from the stroke. For the surgery, they operated on both eyes even though only the right eye appeared off. This was because once my eyes were brought together, my left eye would become a little off-centered. This was just the way the eyes were positioned in my head after my stroke and once one was corrected to a centered position, it was evident that the other eye needed some correction too.

The surgery itself was hard to imagine because it sounded so gross. I was first put to sleep. Then Dr. Brodsky actually cut my eye muscles to tighten and loosen the muscles to adjust the alignment, then they stitched the muscles up. I know it is really hard to imagine having stitches in your eyes, and it was hard for me too! The stitches were probably the worst part of my eye surgery recovery. It was hard to believe I had stitches in my eyes because that is such an unusual place to have stitches. The next day we had to drive to Mayo again for a post-op appointment with the doctor. My eyes were a little sore and the right one especially because they had adjusted two muscles in that eye and only one in the left eye. My eyes definitely felt irritated. It felt like there was sand in my eyes, and I wanted to rub them really badly, but of course I couldn't. The stitches were self-dissolvable, and the doctor said they would feel "crisp." I thought that was a very accurate description even though it sounded awful, but that's what it actually did feel like.

Immediately after the surgery, I had blood in my tears. I wasn't crying. My eyes were wetting themselves from sensing the stitches. The doctor gave me pain medication, but I only took it for a day and a half. Ever since the stroke, which I know was most likely caused by medication, I have been very cautious about taking any medication. They also gave me antibiotic eye drops for four days to prevent infection. After that, I was told to use artificial tears to keep my eyes moist. I also used a greasy gel in my eyes at night for the same purpose. I didn't mind the gel because it felt good, and they told me that applying the gel would lessen the irritating feeling in my eyes and "loosen the stitches." The irritated feeling lasted for about a week, but the redness lasted a very long time! My eyes were very red after the surgery, and they told me to expect that for several weeks; however, it lasted for months.

Luckily, I never experienced double vision, even though the doctor was very confident I would experience it because the deviation was so great. However, as I previously mentioned, because I had an eye misalignment issue when I was little, my brain could better adapt, and therefore, prevent double vision. It was a true blessing. The doctor also told me we would have to wait a couple months "for the smoke to clear" before deciding if another surgery was necessary, and that would be my decision then. I decided almost immediately that I wanted to try again.

My eyes were undoubtedly improved from the surgery, but yet not "perfect." Therefore, I wanted us to try again immediately because I knew I had had such a great doctor who was now familiar with me and my condition. I also was determined to correct my stroke-related physical issues as soon as possible. I had two additional eye surgeries. After the surgeries, I felt my eye looked better, but it was still a little off-center. However, it wasn't off very much, so I was confident my brain would eventually bring my eye in, since it did the same when I was a child. I didn't want to have a fourth surgery and further risk the chances of double vision and any overcorrection. Later, I saw the pictures of my eyes before the first surgery and realized how lucky I was and how improved my eyes actually were.

I also suffered some vision loss after the stroke. I had worn glasses or contacts since I was in kindergarten, but when I was twenty-six and living in Hawaii, I decided to get LASIK. When I inquired about LASIK, I learned that I had very thin corneas, so LASIK wouldn't work for me; however PRK (photo-refractive keratosis) would. This is a different procedure, but it yields similar results to LASIK. I was very nearsighted before I had PRK. When I went to the eye doctor, I could not even see the big /E/ on the chart without my glasses, so I thought I could greatly improve my vision using PRK vision correction. It worked. I no longer needed glasses or contacts, and I could finally wake up in the morning and see without fumbling for my glasses immediately. I thought the change was amazing.

Some might argue my eye surgery was done out of vanity, but without it, I would never see again as others do. Dr. Brodsky even told my parents "For Sara, this isn't a cosmetic issue, it's an identity issue."

There were several instances after my eye surgeries when people didn't notice or comment on them. I thought this was cute because I felt it showed how many people were only seeing the "inside" of me. Of course, I also appreciated positive comments about the surgeries. Mom said they weren't as noticeable as I thought. However, to me, the outcome was incredibly noticeable. I felt so much better after the eye correction. I still had to work on my balance, but somehow I felt bad balance was more socially acceptable than misaligned eyes were. With my eyes fixed, I felt like I was well on my way to the "pre-stroke" Sara. However, due to the stroke, I still lacked depth perception. The loss of depth perception isn't physically noticeable and the only situation where I notice it is when I negotiate a curb or maybe when I exit a restaurant I don't always know if a step is there.

The stroke had also paralyzed my fifth cranial nerve, which controls the jaw and the mouth. As a result, I couldn't open my jaw normally, and when I did open my mouth, it would open crooked. My lower jaw would open to the right. At Northridge Hospital, one time I was trying to eat a banana, and I could not even open my mouth wide enough to eat it. Several months later I tried again, and I could, so I knew my jaw was getting better, although it was still crooked. There was no surgery available to correct my jaw problem, but I wasn't too worried about it because I was the only one who noticed it, and I could tell the use was improving. Even with my jaw, the doctors gave me the same old message, "it just needs more time."

Regardless of all these "time" messages I received from doctors, I stayed very persistent in my stroke recovery. I really felt it was possible to get better, despite the odds against it. I always looked for something miraculous that would be the key to getting me better. I remember one time one of the UWL professors,

Erin Hussey, who was overseeing my therapy, told me she knew I was looking for that "one more thing" because I was always asking her for her opinion on different therapy techniques and theories. It was very true. I knew there had to be some way somehow for me to get better faster.

Despite all my daily therapy, which I knew was helping me get better, it was all much too slow. For me to resume my independent life, I needed to find that "one more thing." My definition of "independence" differs from the therapy world's. In therapy, you are considered "independent" even if you use a walker or a cane, so long as you don't require someone next to you. I described my own "independence" as not requiring any assistive device and no one next to me.

Related to my strong persistence and determination to recover fully, I should expand on my boyfriend at the time. Peter left me. I still don't want to share too many details, but his leaving was emotionally devastating for me. Peter and I had been together for five years, not all after my stroke. The way he stuck by me and supported me for so long after the stroke made his decision to leave me completely shocking. I knew some things he said to me weren't right, but I never mentioned them to family or friends because I didn't want anyone to think badly of him. Still, this omission made it all the more shocking when he left because everyone thought he was a really good guy. He was often critical of me after my stroke and instead of being excited about his visits, I was usually very nervous. He made it clear through his attitude that I would only be welcome back in California with him if I was pretty near perfect. I often specifically had to ask if I looked better on some visits because he would rarely tell me so even though many other people who saw me frequently always complimented me on my progress. I never said anything because

I guess I was just grateful he was with me, and still, everyone always told me how caring and concerned he was.

On the outside, people just saw that he was visiting often and writing nice Caringbridge journals, so he seemed nice, and maybe that's why I didn't receive much support when he left me. We now have zero contact, which is what I prefer. I told him when he left me to never try to come back. I've never regretted saying that. I won't ever speak highly of Peter again. I believe that every nice thing he did for me, he completely nullified by leaving me so suddenly. I remember how he often talked about how difficult my stroke was for him. I am an empathetic person, so I would discuss it with him, but now I reflect back on it all, and I just want to laugh. I was the one who had my life completely turned upside down.

Like everyone else in the world, I was looking for unconditional love. It was heartbreaking to realize that Peter only offered me very conditional love. When I did not meet those conditions in his declared time frame, he simply left me. However, I do wish the best for him, and I hope he's happy. I now realize that he is very superficial and self-centered. Everything has to be perfect for him, on the surface at least, and my disability no longer met his standards. Ours was not a normal break-up. I was seriously disabled, and my so-called "supportive" boyfriend left me because of my disability. It was a horrible feeling, and I'm glad most people won't ever experience it.

Initially I was crushed, but then I surprised myself with my remarkable resilience. I've always been a very independent person, so I was happy to see that trait was still there. I did not let Peter's leaving affect my recovery in any way. I would say, however, that there were a lot of tears the first week, but after that, I started feeling much better. I view the break-up now similarly to how

I view the stroke, an unnecessary and life-altering event, but I can make my peace with both because I'm happy with where my life is now. I'm completely over him, and while I do think less of him for walking out on me, I'm much happier now than I ever would've been with him. I know this is true because I had a dream where I was with Peter (I had no stroke) and when I woke up, I was very relieved it was a dream. I much prefer my reality now. I woke up disabled and alone in Wisconsin, but much happier than I would have been being fine physically with him; I was, however, very surprised and truly disappointed at the lack of support I received after the break-up.

Granted, I had kept all the bad aspects of our relationship secret, but still, my boyfriend left me only due to my disability. I would haveexpected to be greatly supported afterwards at the very least, but I wasn't. The only support I truly felt came from my family, especially my mother.

After Peter left me, two proverbs stuck with me. The first is "you live and learn," and the second is "hindsight is always 20/20." I would consider the latter the key because looking back at that relationship, I really should have been the one who ended it based on relationship problems that were happening that I didn't feel were right. However, to be fair to myself, I did try to end the relationship several times before the stroke. However, Peter was always adamant that we shouldn't end our relationship. When I saw him fighting to stay with me, I conceded and thought if he saw something worth saving for us, maybe I was wrong. This of course brings me to the former proverb that "you live and learn." We all have experiences from different parts of our lives that affect us, but many times all we can do is reflect on our lives and decide how to learn from our mistakes so not to repeat them in the future. In the end, I'm happy that I stuck with Peter because my family really needed a local contact and his help during this terrible time. He did help them greatly in many ways. I'll give him credit for helping my family, but on a personal relationship level, I still had plenty to live and learn from him, which I did.

Nearly four years post-stroke, I found another kind of therapy. Hippotherapy, or horse therapy was my next experimental therapy. This therapy is based on the idea that a horse has a similar gait to a human. By riding a horse, your brain senses this walking motion and rewires. Most important to me, my mom had a good feeling about it. I previously have mentioned how I always believe in my mom's intuition, and this case was no exception. Hippotherapy also can help many other ailments as well—some you would never believe!

I had never been around horses like this, so it was a new experience for me. Riders of all ages and disabilities attended my program at HorseSense. Some riders had autism, some spina bifida, and there was also a class for veterans with PTSD. They had a ramp up to the horse for the disabled rider to mount the horse. I had three helpers: one to lead the horse and one on either side if I needed balance help. Having never ridden a horse before, I requested the "slow, fat, tired horse" and they gave me a beautiful Fjord horse named, Tito. I ended up loving Tito. I participated in this therapy for about a year.

It was right around this time that I began to experience migraines again. I was really disappointed because I hadn't had one since before the stroke, and I was really hoping that I was done with them forever. However, they started again, complete with the dreaded aura. I was very concerned, so I reached out to my neurologist in California, who by this point had also become a friend. He said he could suggest a supplement, but I declined.

I was still being very cautious about what I put in my body, and I knew that most supplements aren't regulated by the FDA. However, I later considered how much this doctor cared about me, and I truly believed he had my best interests at heart, and since I really was concerned about my migraines coming back, I took him up on his offer. He suggested I take 400mg of Riboflavin (B2) daily. I thought this recommendation was relevant to me because I don't eat meat, so I knew I could possibly be deficient in B vitamins. After looking into any contraindications, which I always say is important for everyone when beginning a new medication OR a supplement, I began taking 400mg of Riboflavin. My migraines have significantly been reduced and are very rare now. At most, I've had only a couple a year. If you are a migraine sufferer, consult your doctor to see if this suggestion is okay for you to try.

Wisconsin was a huge step forward in my rehabilitation. I went from the wheelchair to the walker, to the quad cane, to the single-point cane, and eventually to walking unassisted. This progress all occurred in a very familiar environment with family and friends nearby, which I know helped greatly. I am so thankful to have had the support of my family and friends in Wisconsin and their continued love will always mean the world to me.

CHAPTER 18

My Occupational Therapy

THE NEXT THREE chapters discuss my additional daily therapies: Occupational Therapy (OT), Physical Therapy (PT) and Speech Therapy. Occupational Therapy was the least known therapy among my family and friends because what it entails is not obvious from its name. I had never even heard of occupational therapy, until it became a part of my daily life. OT, which largely focuses on arm, hand, and finger movements, was my least favorite of the therapies initially, perhaps because it was definitely the most challenging for me.

The left side of my body was affected the most by the stroke, as it was completely paralyzed for many weeks. However, because my stroke happened in the basilar artery, which is in the brainstem in the middle of the brain, my right side was also severely affected. Tami, my occupational therapist in LaCrosse, said I was her first stroke patient to have significant deficits on both sides of my body—lucky me. With most strokes, typically one side of the body remains unaffected. I am right-handed, so fortunately I was less affected on my right side. I asked Tami what happens when someone's dominant hand is affected, and she said these people quickly change hand dominance to accommodate the deficit. I didn't notice any deficits in my right hand until we did the objective exercise tests in OT. Tami then told me I was weak and slow on both sides. It was much easier and more natural for me to use my right hand because I am right-handed, and my right hand was less affected from the stroke, so of course my therapists wanted me to use my left hand as much as possible to try to return it to normal function. It was incredibly frustrating to use my slow left hand.

Several years after the stroke I was timing an OT task while Peter was visiting. I had him time himself doing the same activity as me and found that my right (my dominant and less affected hand) was slower than his left (non-dominant hand). Subjectively, he said that he felt his left hand was not very good for him. This comparison to Peter made me realize how truly affected both sides of my body were. Even Jen, two years after her stroke incident, told me her hand and arm were still not what they used to be before the stroke, and you can't even tell she ever had a stroke! So, based on Jen's experience, I never expected perfection with my hand either, but I did want to get as close to perfection as I could!

Unfortunately, you cannot solely rely on scheduled therapy for all your recovery. Home exercise is essential, so I would like to review what I did outside of hospital therapy to help my left arm and hand. However, remember this routine did NOT last forever! Three to four days a week I would do 120 triceps lifts with both arms lying in my bed holding a 1 pound dumbbell. I was doing these exercises every day until Tami (thankfully) told me I would benefit more by resting my muscles one day in between. So I began to take a much-desired day off between my "bed exercises."

After using the weight, I used a hand gripper, squeezing it 100 times. Then I would squeeze a therapy clothespin, which had much more resistance than a regular clothespin. I would squeeze the clothespin between my thumb and each of my fingers on both hands 100 times on each hand. The thumb and pinky finger squeeze with my left hand was the most difficult.

Later on, I added a lot of coordination exercises to help my finger dexterity. I didn't enjoy doing these activities, but they were giving me results, so I continued them. I would time myself once a month and record my scores to track my progress. For example, I might time myself using a stopwatch and record how long it took me to take twenty-five Cheerios out of a bowl, one by one. In fact, I often turned to these scores and reviewed them to prove to myself I actually was progressing.

In general, I hated hand coordination exercises. However, my OT therapist always emphasized how important they were, so every day I would do them. I would change the activities often, however, so my body and brain did not get used to doing the identical movements. For example, I would flip a deck of playing cards over with my left hand, stack checkers, put cheerios one by one into a bowl, and place cribbage board pegs into a board and then take them out again, etc. Tami gave me a sheet with a lot of suggestions for hand coordination exercises. I know these exercises probably sound very simple, but for me they were the most challenging, so much so that I would have rather have done a forty-five-minute treadmill workout than stack checkers. Honestly!

I also had a handwriting notebook for penmanship practice. Handwriting was difficult for me because it required a lot of coordination, which I was lacking because of the stroke. After the stroke it was hard to even "hold" a pen due to the paralysis I experienced. I remember I was at Topanga Terrace trying to sign over power of attorney to my mother and I only held the pen and the lawyer positioned the paper against the pen to mark X for my signature. I would date each day in the notebook and within the first couple of months, I saw improvement with my handwriting.

At the beginning, I had a hard time just staying within the lines in my notebook. Actually at first I was just trying to stay between the width of two lines. I still have a notebook from Northridge where the speech therapist drew straight lines on the page with a Sharpie marker. My task was to write my name on the line, but that was very difficult for me.

Jen told me that when she was recovering from her stroke, she started a coordination activity that really helped her. The activity was to touch the tip of each finger to your thumb. Thus, because Jen liked it and it worked for her, I also did this activity countless times for many, many months. I would often do this finger routine when I was walking with my dad. That meant focusing on doing two things at once, which was more challenging than if I were sitting, so I thought it must be more effective. I later abandoned it when a therapist was walking with me and told me that most of the time I wasn't doing the exercise, and I was only making a claw looking position with my hand. This wasn't a message I wanted to send to my brain, so I tried to keep my arms down. I usually awkwardly placed them by my sides at chest level for any reflexes to be ready in case I fell.

Later, I wore my Saebo hand brace which weighted my left arm down and kept my hand flat as it should be. I can still recall the moment when I recognized that my arm reflexes were intact. I was in the living room with my mom on the floor doing therapy exercises. I felt a bug crawling on my right arm, and very quickly, my left arm rose up and brushed the bug away. I know this does not sound like a big deal, but I had not seen my left arm move that fast since I had the stroke. Later, there were many other instances where my left arm came out in front quickly to brace against a fall. For me, it was really exciting to see that my reflexes were still working and my arm could move that fast, even though the movement was only a reflex. It was a good sign of what I was capable of and what I could work up to over time.

Again, as I mentioned previously, I typed this entire book using only my right hand because I wanted to get my story out. Typing this book was not just a physical challenge; it was also emotionally therapeutic. It was important to sit down and try to accomplish putting my thoughts and memories down both for myself and to share with others.

One of the most difficult, yet important, therapies for me was typing. Typing was very difficult for me with only my right hand available to use; my left hand was very slow at the time. I was surprised how few people mentioned typing as being that difficult post-stroke because it was certainly frustrating for me. My guess is that this was possibly related to age. I was young enough to have accepted the computer and email as an important form of communication. Older generations, who more often experience strokes, may not have embraced the computer and email as much as I had. But for me, typing was certainly where I immediately noticed my hand deficits from the stroke. In fact, I suggest if you know a stroke survivor, rethink the use of email for communication. Using the phone for contacting caregivers is much easier. Just try typing an email one-handed, and you'll see how difficult it is. Typing requires a lot of finger dexterity, something I knew was greatly lacking then.

Practicing typing every day didn't help me improve even a single minute on my set typing practice exercise. What did help was doing more and more coordination tasks, and of course, a lot of time. I'm not suggesting doing less therapy because I'm a believer in therapy, but I do think I would have better spent my time doing coordination tasks other than typing. I needed to improve my finger dexterity in order to improve my typing, and it was the coordination tasks that helped me do that, not typing. Using both hands to type was much more time-consuming and frustrating than only using my right hand, believe it or not. Using one hand was frustrating, but it did help me to communicate my thoughts and my small achievements. I honestly don't think I would've written this book if I had forced myself to use two hands to type it.

Other OT tasks that I did at home were: playing the piano (I played as a child, but it was incredibly difficult after the stroke), washing dishes, lifting dumbbells, pulling cans from the cabinet shelf and then putting them back, etc.

I absolutely hated counting exercise repetitions in my head. Of course, you do have to do it in order to keep track. However, I would always lose my focus while counting because I had to focus so hard on the exercise at hand. To try to keep track I would hold out the fingers on my right hand. I would also try to think of a special significance for the numbers. This sometimes made counting easier, so if I forgot the number, I would think, *Did I think of that person?* Sometimes I would remember the person instead of the number. I used birthdays the most. For example, my birthday is August 7, so when I would get to 7, I would think *my birthday*. Sometimes this association would help, and sometimes it wouldn't. Or, I would say the number out loud, if possible, and sometimes that would help. The best way was if someone was with me, and my parents often were, and then I would have them help me count. But I would still count in my head, and a good thing I did because sometimes they were off too or weren't doing it! However, if I lost track, I could at least ask, *What number are we on?* Often they could tell me, which I loved because it was much better than guessing.

My first OT worked with me while I was at the nursing home, Topanga Terrace. Her name was Olga. Olga came from Romania. When I was little, I loved my VHS tape of the Olympic gold medalist, the Romanian gymnast Nadia Comaneci. I loved it so much that I wore the tape out from watching it every day. Because I watched it so often, my family was very familiar with Nadia too. I wanted to be a gymnast just like Nadia one day. Nadia is also from Romania, so my family and I felt we had a connection to Romania via this video. Olga worked with me the whole time I was at Topanga. I remember one time when I was working with Olga and I knew that I would be moving to Northridge, I asked her, "How long do you think it will be until my left hand is better?" I was always obsessed with "how long?" questions. Because Olga had worked with me for so long, I figured she could be the best judge of my arm and hand ability.

"Sara, you need a lot of acute rehab," she responded. Obviously no one wants to hear their therapist say they still need "a lot of acute rehab," but I appreciated her honesty.

Olga worked very hard with me. In therapy, you are normally given a certain number of patients to work with each day, and when you are done working with these patients, you may leave. So if Olga worked longer, which she often did with me, she did so voluntarily on her extra time. That was so generous of her. She has the sweetest voice and was always so encouraging with me. My parents loved her because she was kind and gentle.

One time Dad remembered having a dream, and he retold it to Olga. In the dream, I "slugged" him. Olga told Dad "I don't think she's far away!" Later that day, back in my room, I was in my bed, and my parents were sitting on the right side of me, when my mom asked, "Sara do you want to slug your father?" I was very slowly moving my right arm back, and so I slowly lowered it to "slug" dad, with help from Mom guiding me. We all had a good laugh. It wasn't really a slug—it was more of a tap—yet it was an arm movement that I must say did vaguely resemble a "slug." I guess it made Dad's dream come to life a bit for all of us and for us to see that my recovery WAS happening, even though in this situation I required assistance from Mom.

Another OT therapist from Topanga that I worked with was Mylah. Mylah is originally from The Philippines, so she speaks Tagalog as well as English. Because I love languages, I saw our interaction as a learning opportunity. I would try to learn Tagalog phrases from her. When I was doing my therapy with Mylah, I often forgot which number I was on in my repetitions, so she would ask "Bonus Sara?" I would reply in Tagalog "Hindi bonus, Mylah!" which in English means "No bonus, Mylah!" She enjoyed my interest in Tagalog and also how much of the language I could remember. I was happy to see that my interest in other languages remained and was helping me exercise my brain a bit. I'm upset with myself for not taking advantage of more language practice with Olga, from Romania. I imagine this is because I was non-verbal when I began working with Olga. Because Mylah couldn't arrive until evenings most days, she would come to my room.

Sometimes my "therapy" exercise would entail getting me ready for bed. I enjoyed this exercise because it was functional. Providing functional activities is something I also strived to do as a teacher, using authentic materials and activities in the classroom. Students always respond well to anything we practice in the classroom that they can directly apply to their real world. I felt the same about therapy. So in my OT session, I would brush my teeth and put on face cream, which I would do anyway at home. It doesn't sound like much, but it actually requires a lot of work with your hands and taking off and putting on all the caps, etc. Brushing your teeth is also a lot of OT work. I had many great occupational therapists at Topanga, but Olga and Mylah worked with me the most often. When I would fall asleep, I would try to do so lying on my left side because in therapy I remembered they did "weight bearing" activities to try to build strength in my left side. Although not the same thing exactly, I thought maybe it would yield similar results if I put my weight on my left side while sleeping.

When I arrived at Northridge, I met my occupational therapist named Mia, the very next morning around 8 a.m. I was still in bed. Mia entered the room and said, "You're so adorable! Now how many people can be told that straight out of bed?" I smiled because it was a very sweet thing for Mia to say. She helped me change out of my hospital gown and into my clothes for the day, which was good practice and actually very challenging OT for me. I told Mia I liked that kind of activity, again because it was functional, something I could then do every day. Mia was my primary occupational therapist at Northridge, although I worked with many others as well while I was there. Carole was one of them. She nicknamed me Sara "Patience" because I tended to be very impatient with some things. My parents remembered this name and also often called me Sara "Patience" in Wisconsin when they wanted me to be especially patient with something.

I also remember Mia telling me "You have the longest arms ever!" This was actually bad because I always wanted to reach out to grab for stability instead of walking closer to hold on to something. I thought it was more stable to reach out, but actually it was more unsafe for me to do that. So sometimes Dad would say, "Sara, let's make this a non-reaching day!" I didn't want to reach either, but it was a natural reaction and very hard to break.

At Northridge they called me a "feeder" because I needed someone to feed me my food. I didn't have enough movement in my arms and hands for the first several months after my stroke to feed myself. Someone had to be with me and literally feed me my food. The nurses usually helped feed me breakfast, while my parents helped with lunch and dinner. In OT, we even practiced opening packets one day. My dad also remembers that whenever I would grab a glass to drink, I would bring it really fast to my face. I would do the same with a fork or spoon. I still did not have much coordination or control of the speed and accuracy of my limbs. To accommodate my lack of control while eating, I was always assisted with the food.

I remember not being able to do many things with my hands for months. As an example, at Topanga, I was lying in bed once, and I felt way too warm. I wanted to take a blanket off my legs, but I couldn't do it. Around the same time, my dad was trying to have me throw a ball to him and I couldn't release the ball.

My hand would just come down and hit the bed, but with the ball still there in it. This was even using my dominant and less affected right hand. I also remember not being able to press the nurse button or use the remote for the TV because it was too difficult for me to press. I knew all these things were very easy, but I just couldn't do them yet.

My occupational therapist in Wisconsin, Tami, however, saw me do many things with my hands for the first time after the stroke because a lot of time had passed since the stroke when she became my therapist. I started working with Tami at seven months after the stroke. One day for therapy, we sat on a mat table. For our therapy session, Tami had brought medical scrub clothes for me to put on over my own clothes. During that OT session, I also tied my shoes alone for the first time after the stroke. I know that does not sound like much, but in therapy it is a big deal when you can tie your own shoes. Later, I also had to retrain myself on how to zip my jacket, button my pants and shirt, and put my hair in a ponytail holder. When my dad saw me tie my shoes, he said "I'm surprised you can do that already, Sara!"

"I'm not," Tami said immediately.

I was pleasantly surprised too because I remembered trying this same skill with Mia at Northridge and failing. Also, at Topanga, Olga skipped having me attempt to tie my shoes because it was too advanced for me. Tying shoes is something that not everyone can do again after a stroke, so I knew I was on the right track at least.

At night when I slept, I wore a big, clunky brace on my left hand because my left hand always wanted to curl into a fist. The brace was meant to train my brain to keep my fingers and hand flat and not develop the curled hand, wrist and arm deficit that unfortunately many stroke patients acquire. My mom had heard about the brace from a work colleague, so she definitely asked about the brace immediately when we started my therapy in Wisconsin. My brace was made by Saebo. You do need to have someone certified in Saebo to fit you for the brace, like my therapist, Tami. Tami thought I was very borderline for needing the brace because I had sufficient hand movement; however, she also thought I still might benefit from it. Despite my "borderline" status, after several months, Tami definitely did note a difference in the relaxation of my hand, as did Mom. Initially, I was scared of the brace because I remembered the foot drop boots I wore that hurt every time I woke up. However, I had no similar issues with the Saebo.

The Saebo looks like an open glove, which your hand just slides into and then is held flat with Velcro straps. Best of all, I could remove the brace if it hurt, and fortunately it never did. I didn't mind the brace, and if people thought it helped my hand, then even better! Ultimately, Tami and my family were very happy that I wore the brace at night to help relax my hand and fingers into a more natural state. Even later when I stopped wearing the brace, I stayed very diligent to try to always fall asleep with my hand flat under my body.

There is a phenomenon called left or right arm "neglect." This is when a stroke patient rehabs their arm into what they feel is sufficient function. However, since it isn't to an acceptable level of function for the body, the body will "neglect" it and it becomes useless. I was not willing to let this happen. I got really tired of hearing from my family, "Left hand!" They wanted me to do everything with my left hand. I remember one time I was zipping up my jacket to go to therapy, and my dad saw me hold the bottom of my jacket with my right hand, and zip the jacket with my left hand, which is harder for coordination. Seeing this, he gave me a kiss on the cheek, and I thought to myself, only my dad would think I would deserve a kiss on the cheek for that! I was very unhappy with my left hand because it was so slow to respond, hesitant in its movements and very inaccurate and unable to complete many small tasks. However, because everyone wanted my left hand to improve so badly, they would often nag me about it and want me to add more rehab tasks. I would cry sometimes because I felt I was already doing too much rehab, and I felt it was mentally unsafe to add any more exercises to my already full-time routine. I would think to myself, *Can't I just rest for a minute? I've already done so much today!*

Tami wanted me to "balance" my days with more arms and less legs, but I was very resistant to that idea because I didn't want my walking to be delayed at all. Walking was my primary goal, and I was very honest about it. Before the stroke, I rarely had done any exercises for my upper body and arms. So Tami and I now joked that maybe this was my "exercise karma." The stroke gave me no options. I had to do arm exercises. Before the stroke, I had totally ignored my arms at the gym. No way was I going to be satisfied now with my weak, slow hand, and arm post-stroke. My goal was to get it back to normal as much as possible, so I began paying closer attention to my arm exercises.

Tami has four sisters, and she told me one of them was on the birth control pill. I urged Tami to discuss the Pill with her sister and encourage her to stop taking it. Tami did, and her sister stopped. I was very happy to hear that because my goal since the stroke has always been to warn women of the potential dangers of hormonal birth control, and urge them to have more detailed conversations with their doctors, so they will avoid taking combined estrogen and progesterone birth control if they experience migraines with aura. Remember, progesterone-only birth control is the "safest." I know I would never have used it at all had I known what the result would be and how much rehab time I would have to put in to get better. So with that said, I spread my cautionary tale in hopes I can help save lives by educating women that what happened to me (a young healthy person), could happen to anyone.

One thing that was especially frustrating was the constant unfairness I encountered in my therapy. I know there is nothing "fair" about having a stroke at age twenty-seven and missing out on years of your life, but I also struggled with unfairness in my therapy. Let me be clearer. For my occupational therapy, I would practice coordination exercises and then time myself on the same activity monthly and record my scores to track my progress. You would think that "fair" would only be to get better. However, almost every month, something would get worse. I would think *How is that possible?* I've practiced for hours, and so much time has passed, and I've only gotten worse? Then Dr. Stacey Meardon, a professor at the University of Wisconsin-LaCrosse (UWL) at the time, told me this was completely normal and is actually a sign the brain is reorganizing and trying to rewire. I said, "So it's a good sign?" "I guess" she replied.

I have always been a positive person, so I decided then to interpret these frustrating situations as "good signs" to maintain my motivation. I also tried to find new activities to add to my routine to bust through any plateaus and to get better. I felt my brain was bored sometimes, and it needed new activities to continue to be challenged. I was really happy that I could document my times so I could see a positive trend in the reduction of my timing of tasks, even when some activities were slower.

I had certain theories about OT. The first was that multitasking OT and PT is beneficial. I described how I did this when walking for physical therapy and I simultaneously touched my thumb and fingertips together, but then I realized that I was creating a bad hand position so I stopped doing this. In the end, I don't think this theory is actually true. Another idea I had was that healing the coordination center in my brain would also help heal the damaged balance center in my brain. While healing my coordination undoubtedly helped me, I don't think it helped my balance in any real way. Regular walking and countless other balance activities helped that aspect.

Another theory I had was that there is only an X amount of therapy you can do in a day. I did a lot of therapy daily, but I didn't want to feel like I should constantly be doing therapy. I did hours of therapy, and when I was done, I was done for that day. I also used this view as an excuse if someone wanted to nag me about doing more therapy. I would say, "I've already done X hours of therapy today." I don't know if this theory is true or not, but I always went by it. I think quite simply that time is extremely important and shouldn't be overlooked. This of course means including some rest time! You're welcome, stroke patients! It has to be a mix of therapy and rest. Neither therapy alone nor rest alone will help you improve. It has to be both.

CHAPTER 19

Give Me a Hand (OT continued)

Y INSURANCE STOPPED paying for my therapy visits, so I financially had to stop attending scheduled therapy. Later I was very fortunate to be able to attend physical and occupational therapy sessions with therapy students and professors at the university of Wisconsin-LaCrosse (UWL).

We thought this solution was a great way around the insurance. We were very fortunate to be able to attend therapy there, and they felt they were very fortunate to have me there as a learning example for the students. I think the professors were aware how rare it is to have someone my age suffer from a stroke, and they knew I would be a great learning opportunity for the students. Although older than the students, I was still closer in age to them than to the professors so I felt they bonded with me through the therapy and really wanted me to get better. Also, it is always good to have an objective eye watching you do your exercises.

I first attended occupational therapy at UWL in early 2011. The two girls who first worked with me wanted to introduce me to constraint-induced movement therapy (CIMT) and modified constraint-induced movement therapy (mCIMT), which we finally settled on doing. This idea involves using the affected limb in a variety of activities while the unaffected limb is restrained in a sling or mitt. Modified CIMT is the same thing, just for a shorter period—two hours vs. six hours every day. I know that it doesn't sound difficult, but for me, nothing sounded worse. To attempt to describe the difficulty of this activity, I told my friends to imagine doing these exercises with their non-dominant hand, but then make it at least twenty times more difficult because they weren't stroke victims. In retrospect, that was too generous. It was much more difficult.

CIMT was a therapy I had heard about, but I was not excited to try it because it involved my left (more affected) hand so much. However, I was curious about it and also highly motivated to get my left hand better so I gave it my best shot. I did two hours of fifteen-minute occupational therapy tasks every day for two weeks. In the end, I had good results! The therapists administered the Jebsen Hand Function Test (JHFT) test to observe my pre- and post-test results. Not only did I improve on their exam, but I also did on my own scores I was keeping at home AND my typing which I was more than pleased to see. However, the "unrealistic goals" side of me had expected much more dramatic results. When I told people about the therapy, they often asked

"Why not just continue since you're getting results?" While this question is understandable, it's almost laughable from a stroke sufferer's point of view because using the affected limb is always so frustrating. No, this therapy is not feasible long term.

Another thing I noticed is the saying "It's hard, frustrating, difficult, challenging" never was a legitimate excuse. However, I must say, any time you hear these words from a stroke patient, listen to them. Imagine one of your limbs falling asleep and then your being told to do some fine coordination activities. "It's hard" often means, "It's impossible," or "how absurd of you to ask me." I never experienced the pins and needles feeling, but that is the closest I can come to making it relatable for a non-stroke patient. I felt that my frustration after the stroke was incredibly amplified. I think stroke patients should be given a break sometimes, especially when something they are doing may not seem so difficult to someone else. Still, it can be terribly frustrating to a stroke patient.

I tried to do everything I could with only my right hand because it was so much more difficult to use my left hand. For example, I would open a piece of candy in a wrapper by biting on one twisted end and pulling the candy out of the wrapper with my teeth and right hand. When I wanted to apply Chapstick, I would bite off the cap instead of using my left hand, and then use my right hand to apply it. Or, when I put on glasses, I would use my right hand to straighten out the frames on the right side and my face to push out the left side. In my defense, I knew there was a way I could actually tie my shoes with one hand, but I purposely never learned it because I knew I'd use it if I knew it. As I became better with my left hand, I incorporated it more. However, it took hours and years of therapy.

About four years after my stroke, I created a new occupational therapy for myself, which I named Sara-py after myself. Sara-py was what I originally thought constraint- induced movement therapy (CIMT) was. It basically forces the use of the affected limb; however, the other hand isn't restrained because I needed it for balance. I thought that was silly if I was motivated enough to create this new therapy for myself.

Instead of just focusing on certain tasks for a set number of hours, Sara-py is incorporating the affected limb as much as possible throughout the entire day. For example, to brush my teeth, I'd take the cap of the toothpaste off with my left hand, brush with my left hand and adjust the water with my left hand. However, unlike CIMT, there were no tedious tasks to do. Still, since this was an all-day every-day occurrence, I encountered many more coordination challenges than I had ever faced with CIMT. Best of all, without all the tedious little coordination tasks, it felt more like real life. Remember, however, that I am in NO way a therapist, so please don't consider Sara-py to be a valid form of therapy that you should use. However, I do recommend creating your own schedule for therapy because I think it can give you motivation.

When I first tried Sara-py, four years post-stroke, I lasted a couple of weeks until I decided it was too advanced and over-whelming for me. However, the idea stayed in the back of my mind. Then, a year and a half later, I tried it again. It still wasn't easy, but not as overwhelming as before, so I kept it up for a longer period. A couple of months in, I really regretted not taking any pre-test scores because I had no way to objectively measure my progress. While I vaguely thought I could see a difference, as I previously stated, stroke progress is very slow and subtle, so it was nearly impossible for me to identify my progress subjectively. I liked Sara-py, the second time around anyway, mainly because while it was super challenging, I was still able to personalize it and set the rules because it was my own idea. However, it IS advanced, and it showed me once again, that regardless of exercise intensity, time is still so important for rehab. Like most OT tasks, I again abandoned it when I grew sick of it. However, I continued other OT activities and also returned to Sara-py occasionally.

I also began to notice a person's hand dominance. I was constantly paying the most attention to left hand exercises to get better, so I was especially secretly happy when I noticed a left-handed individual. I was amazed at how easily these people used their left hands. I focused on movies, TV, real life, whenever and wherever! Not intently, I only recognized my increased awareness. The closest left-handed individual to me is my mother. However, I also watched my dad sometimes because he's also right-handed like me, and I noticed whenever he naturally used his left hand.

I ended up visiting a local gym called "The Wellness Center" at Vernon Memorial Hospital (VMH) in Viroqua, Wisconsin, a short drive from Westby, where I lived. I knew my arms especially were very weak and could benefit from weight training. I had thought my arms were weak before the stroke too, so I was really nervous to see where I was with my arm strength after the stroke. I went to the Wellness Center because it is the closest gym near Westby, and I had visited the Wellness Center pre-stroke, so I was familiar with the gym and the staff. I had never tried the arm equipment before at any gym, so this was a new experience and I had no memory to measure it against. I remember using the pectoral fly/chest machine and not being able to lift any weight. I could only use the bar. I didn't perform impressively on the other machines, but I could at least use a weight. However, I eventually built up my arm strength to what the therapists called "normal." I was very happy to be able to use the Wellness Center to build my strength again.

My first group of occupational therapy students at UWL administered an occupational therapy survey to me. This questionnaire is designed to assess the survivors' use of their affected limb. You give yourself a ranking depending on the question for how well you perform a certain activity, such as opening doors, carrying something, etc. I remember thinking I could almost rank everything as never having used my non-dominant hand like that before the stroke. I thought, *Was I really that right-hand dominant?* Then I remembered a time in Los Angeles pre-stroke where I was eating in a restaurant with my boyfriend at the time. We were both right-handed, but I noticed he would hold his fork in his left hand and cut with his right hand, so he could use the fork to eat with his left hand. I would start this same way so I could cut with my right hand, but then I would switch silverware, so I could also eat with my right hand. I tried to assimilate to his style which was actually more efficient and "correct," but it was too difficult, so I quickly reverted back to my old way of eating. This memory made me realize that I was, in fact, very right-hand dominant before the stroke.

The following fall semester, I attended UWL again with a new class and new therapists. These new occupational therapy students introduced a new therapy to me—mirror therapy, which was fairly new in the occupational therapy world. In this therapy, you use a large mirror to focus on while you do movements with the unaffected arm, which your brain interprets as being two hands. You are focusing on the hand in the mirror while doing the same movement with the affected hand behind the mirror. That is supposed to trick your brain and rewire your brain in the same way it would if you really did have two unaffected hands. I thought it sounded like a very interesting therapy. Like the students, I was excited to try it. I performed mirror therapy for thirty minutes per day for five weeks.

When I started mirror therapy, the students gave me a research article, which I appreciated. They also gave me a checklist, so I could mark when I did mirror therapy each day and for how long. I really liked this idea too because it made me more accountable. Subjectively, I felt I was getting better because later on, I had to add activities to meet the thirty-minute time requirement that was set. However, the day we had to retest, I also had to retest my home OT scores that day, and they weren't the greatest, so I entered the session that day feeling kind of nervous. I told the girls that my scores that morning weren't the greatest to prepare them for the worst. I also wanted their professor to explain any bad scores. I didn't want them to enter the workforce after graduating feeling disheartened after seeing my potential road bumps after all their hard work. In the end, my scores did improve, and I was, of course, very happy to see that happen.

One way I was able to see my progress subjectively was to hate things less. I don't like saying that I hated things, but I did then. I remember once the UWL girls said I "liked" fine motor activities because they knew I was doing them at home. I told them, "Let's be clear, I don't 'like' these activities. I do them because I think they're helping me get better." I never "liked" an OT activity, but I could tell when I didn't mind the things as much, and I thought that was great.

Occupational therapy was incredibly challenging for me. My therapist, Tami, also emphasized how repetition was so very important, which often made many occupational therapy exercises monotonous and boring. I guess persistence is the key with occupational therapy, no matter how frustrating it becomes. In my situation, where progress was always so hard for me to see, it would have been very easy to give up. However, I kept my end goal in mind, and with every repetition I would think to myself, *That's one less I'll have to do before I'm "normal" again.* I knew I had to have both hands working to reach my ultimate goal of normalcy, and that thought kept me going day by day.

CHAPTER 20

Physical Therapy

PHYSICAL THERAPY (PT) also played a huge role in my recovery. While occupational therapy generally focuses on the waist up, physical therapy focuses on the waist down. My stroke greatly affected the balance center in my cerebellum, so suddenly I was unable to walk. Imagine that your ability to walk disappears in an instant. Before the stroke, I never would have guessed how much balance is required for actual walking and so many other functions in life, but I certainly came to know how essential balance is to live your daily life.

For a while, I had to rely on a wheelchair to get around. Yet I only saw the wheelchair as temporary. I had every intention of graduating from it as quickly as possible. In fact, I saw my entire disability as being only "temporary," it just ended up being a longer-term "temporary" than I would have ever imagined. All things considered, I was lucky, as many people in wheelchairs never have the ability to graduate from it. However, I was confident that I would eventually get out of the wheelchair, and so was everyone around me. That confidence definitely helped me mentally feel more assured and even more determined.

My regular physical therapists at Topanga were Patti and Becky. I later learned that Patti rarely ever saw patients because she was as busy with administrative duties as the head of rehab, so I felt very privileged having her as my therapist. I remember often lying on a mat table in the rehab room and my physical therapist for the day was Patti or Becky who asked me "Sara, can you move ___?" I wondered, *Why is everyone so interested in me moving, and why are they so excited when I do?* I didn't understand what was going on then. I could not move much at all. However, I remember it being a really big deal for everyone when I could move anything. I started by moving a few fingers, and then inch-by-inch, a bit more movement returned to my limbs over months of time and trying. I even remember my parents calling my family back home and telling them what I actually could move. I didn't think it was all worth calling home about, but they sure did.

Weeks later, Becky even took a picture of me on my back raising my legs slightly and holding them up in the air for the first time. She later showed me that picture when I was at Northridge when she and Patti visited. Patti and Becky were the first to get my muscles moving again after the stroke, for which I am so grateful. For my "birthday present" on August 7, 2009, two months after my stroke, Patti let me stand using the standing machine, and it holds you in place. Just standing up at that time was ambitious, but Patti and Becky were also there, so I could hang on to them. After lying down for so many weeks, my body had seemingly stretched out, so much so that Dad said it looked like I had grown taller. I am 5'8" and Patti is 5'10", but Dad said we seemed about the same height. I did not notice any difference, but much later during a doctor's visit, they did measure my height and I was still only 5'8".

As weeks turned into months, I even "walked" for the first time again at Topanga. It was with a walker. My left hand was velcroed to the walker, when I attempted those steps, and my therapist, Becky, was down on the ground helping me place my feet, each one in front of the other. When I completed the session, I told Sharon, the administrator, that I was ready to go home because she had said I could leave the nursing home when I could walk. She just laughed. I still required too much assistance, but she was so proud that I was upright and starting to walk. I wasn't impressed because I needed so much assistance, but my parents were excited, walker assistance and all. It was a solid sign to them that I was slowly recovering, and that the therapy was working.

At Topanga, I realized I had two special physical challenges to overcome—subluxation and clonus. My therapist said my shoulders were "subluxed." Basically this meant that my shoulders would slip out of their sockets occasionally. This was because I had been bedridden for so long, and therefore, I lost muscle mass as I was unable to move. To remedy my subluxation, they would tape my arms with kinesio-tape to try to keep them in place. They then began cleansing my skin with a cotton ball soaked in rubbing alcohol to rid my skin of any lotion or leftover tape. Then they cut and carefully positioned the tape to secure my shoulders. They also taped the outside of my arms to my upper shoulders to try to hold them in place. The therapist would re-tape me every few days. I remember during my last month at Topanga, the therapist who was taping my arms had me actually feel the half-inch gap between my arm and arm socket. Because of that subluxation, they also attached a tray to my wheelchair so I could rest my elbows on it and not have my arms dangle to the sides and cause more downward pressure on my shoulders. I hated that tray because I thought it made the wheelchair look like a high chair. The taping of my shoulders only occurred at Topanga, and after a few weeks of the tape, my shoulders were stronger. I still was so weak that I could not hold my head up, so I was constantly braced with towels around my neck or my parents held my head up. My mom convinced Patti that she needed to use ultrasound treatments followed by muscle massage. This description sounded more like a massage, rather than therapy, so they had some skepticism, but after a short time I was able to hold my head up without support and then move my head from left to right by myself.

I also suffered from clonus. That was when my ankle would in-voluntarily shake up and down very fast for no apparent reason. To make my foot and ankle stop the repeated shaking, I would either reposition my foot or hold my leg down with my right hand. My mom thought my body was just shaking to "wake myself up." I still don't know why I developed clonus because I have never experienced it before, but it was one more thing I had to deal with post-stroke. Unlike subluxation, clonus was a condi-tion that followed me after Topanga. Therapists could identify what it was, but everyone else around me usually looked at me weirdly when my leg started shaking for no apparent reason. I also noticed it happened more when I was tired, like when I was at the gym, for example. It still occurs today.

In PT at Topanga the therapists began to use "electrode therapy" on me. The therapists placed electrodes on different locations of my body. First using water, the therapists removed the excessive lotion the CNAs always rubbed on me to keep my skin moisturized. Then the electrodes were plugged into a machine that looked like an old tape cassette player. The electrodes themselves are just round discs that stick to your skin and are attached to a cord, which is then plugged into the machine. When turned on, the machine sends a light electrical pulse through your body and your muscles involuntarily move. The purpose is to help your brain recognize the muscles that were now unfamiliar to my body and brain, which I couldn't move.

Although the therapy sounds odd, I was encouraged to learn it was originally designed to help the former professional skier, Picabo Street, who was injured in a skiing accident. Since the electrodes sent little shocks that jolted the skin, I thought there was a good chance that the jolts would also "wake me up" out of the nightmare that I thought I was in. Before realizing that I had actually had a stroke, I remember thinking it was odd when the therapists called for the "stroke protocol." The electrodes didn't hurt. It was just annoying having to stay still for fifteen to twenty minutes and have a bit of electric current run through my body, involuntarily twitching my muscles.

At Northridge my physical therapists were Molly and Janelle. Molly had been a part of the therapy program at Northridge Hospital for years. Janelle was a physical therapy student about to graduate, and she was working as an intern to satisfy a requirement for her university. Molly and Janelle worked very hard with me. At Northridge, I was walking in the hallways using a wall railing and then a walker. I became obsessed with how long it was going to take me to get better. I would beg them not to send me home in a wheelchair. They assured me they were doing everything they could to help me walk. Weeks later, I did go home in a wheelchair, but that was only because of how severe my stroke was, not any reflection on the quality of my therapy. Molly and Janelle always worked very hard with me in the therapy room and used various exercises and machines to help me build back my strength. They were also the first therapists to take me to "pool therapy."

When I arrived back in Wisconsin from California, I had to wait over a month to even begin therapy due to the insurance red tape. Because of this issue, I began my own therapy at home. I can't say enough good things about my parents and their dedication to doing therapy with me. In fact, I think my Dad deserves an honorary physical therapy degree because he worked with me so much as my therapist. Every day, Dad would come over and help oversee my therapy routine for the day. Often, I would get up, and he would assist me to walk around the nearby high school track or inside my mom's house. Then I would return home to have breakfast, followed by some coordination exercises and forty-five minutes on the treadmill. Mom helped me with everything else, my meals, bathing, dressing, midnight trips to the bathroom, etc. They are both truly remarkable people, and I'm so honored to have them in my life. I don't know how I was so lucky to have these amazing parents.

We decided to get a treadmill because there is a lot of research that supports the use of a treadmill for faster stroke recovery. I would always beg to go faster or longer on the treadmill. Dad was a great physical therapist. He worked with me for so many months that he could quickly tell when I was off balance, and he knew all my walking issues. He would often say "Left foot straight! Point your left hip! Small steps!" etc. Not at the same time but only when applicable, which was often. I actually liked it when he "coached" me as he would tell me if I was walking well or poorly because I couldn't see it myself. I mean, I could tell if I stumbled, but that was about it. Starting out, I used the walker, and Dad would always say "Left hand on the walker!" I had a hard time just keeping my left hand on the walker because my grip was so weak. Dad was really happy when I accepted the walker as help because he also saw it as temporary and the first step toward getting rid of the wheelchair.

Dad would ask me daily "Are you tired?" However, I never knew how to answer the question. I didn't know if he meant physically tired or mentally tired, so I think I may have answered him inconsistently at times. For example, I would get physically tired after my forty-five minutes on the treadmill, but mentally tired after walking just one lap at the track. Therefore, I liked the treadmill much more than walking at the track because I didn't have to concentrate on balance so much on the treadmill. On the treadmill, I could simply hang onto the handrails. At the track, I was holding on to nothing, so I needed to have absolute focus on every step. In fact, I remember initially thinking about the idea of walking around the track and that idea alone with nothing to hang on to was very intimidating. However, I always wore a gait belt around my waist, and Dad always kept hold of some part of it just in case I fell.

Dad and I would often go to the high school track when school was out for the summer. The track was quiet then. My first time around the track took a ridiculously long time for me to walk. I clocked in at 57 minutes, and I used a quad cane the last 100 meters. However, we kept trying, day after day. I liked the track much more than walking inside at my mom's house because there were less turns I had to make, and it was really nice to be outside. It was also easy to see how far we had walked. Kathy, my physical therapist at the time, told us not to keep track of the time. However, we thought it was encouraging to see my time going down, so we continued doing that. We were really disappointed when winter arrived in Wisconsin and we could no longer use the outdoor track for our walking, until spring.

I also often heard that I should have "realistic expectations." However, I always disagreed with this idea. Yes, I had very unrealistic expectations and they often left me disappointed time-wise because my recovery was so long. However, more importantly, my expectations gave me stronger motivation. If I said "Okay, realistically I want to be able to walk one lap at the track in thirty minutes," I would have met that goal easily and then what? Stop rehabbing because I met my realistic goal? No way would I EVER have done that. So I preferred my long-range lofty goals, which I basically knew were unattainable. So, I was never disappointed with my short-term therapy progress (of course after I learned and accepted how slow progress after a stroke really is). Instead, I took what I could get and was happy with all I could achieve.

Complimenting me in the beginning was a dangerous thing. I had very thin skin and a compliment early on meant I looked odd and stood out, so I would cry. Fortunately, I developed a "thicker skin," so attempts to commend me were appreciated. Even the rare and rude comment, "What's wrong with her?" stopped bothering me. Then, I began to really appreciate the compliments and wondered why they had bothered me before. It took a long time, however, to get to the point where I could accept and appreciate compliments. Sometimes, I felt like the therapists didn't want to compliment me because they felt like they were overdoing it. However, when I was blind to my progress, I really needed and appreciated the comments to keep me going.

An exercise that Dad had me do right after we arrived home from California was just standing with my walker. Initially, I was very afraid to walk for fear of falling, so Dad would have me stand with the walker for ten to twenty minutes because standing was the first step to walking. As you can imagine, it was very boring. To make it a little more interesting, he placed the walker in front of the TV, so that I would be distracted somewhat. I would try to lean on my left side more, because that was my weaker side, and I thought doing that might strengthen it. I quickly learned that it was very difficult to maintain my balance standing whenever something around me was moving—whether it was a motion on the TV or our cat walking across the floor, or a commotion outside the window. Any of these motions would throw off my focus and in turn throw off my balance. I later learned that this happened because my stroke occurred in the cerebellum, which is responsible for movement and vision, thus hampering my balance.

Because of the connection between movement, vision, and the cerebellum, I developed another hypothesis. I often stumbled or fell off-balance as well when I heard something. My theory was that since vision affected me due to the stroke occurring in my cerebellum, I theorized that sound waves, on a much smaller level, were also moving items. This could explain why noises threw me off. However, my physical therapists attributed it more to distractions than to sound waves.

Dad would always complain that I lacked focus. I thought that was kind of funny because my friend I met in Hawaii, Cary, used to tease me about just the opposite trait. One morning, when I was living in Hawaii, Cary, her son Kai, and I were walking to a restaurant to eat breakfast. We were walking on the sidewalk, and a truck drove by us with what Cary describes as a "giant Hawaiian flag" hanging out the window. When the truck passed us, Cary asked, "Wow, did you see that flag?" I responded, "What flag?" I had completely missed it. Cary then asked "How could you have missed it? That flag was huge!" From then on, Cary would always tease me about being overly focused on the task at hand and never getting distracted. Because of that scenario, I thought it was ironic, even funny, that one of my issues post-stroke was that I was too easily distracted. However, I still struggle with noticing things. I think this is just a "Sara-thing."

Early on in my stroke rehab, I also had issues post-stroke with "impulsivity." For example, when I would take a drink of water, I would bring the glass to my mouth much too quickly. Or if I saw something that I needed, I would reach for it without thinking in advance if I would knock something else over to get it. Everyone around me complained that I did everything too fast and with too much impulse.

I want to describe my walking progression here. I began with the walker, then I moved to the quad cane (a four-point cane), then to a single-point cane, then to no device at all. However, I ended up returning to the walker and staying there for a while because I felt more secure with it, and the walker also gave me the most independence. When I began walking alone with no device (but still someone holding my gait belt from behind, nothing in my hand), you might think that I would be really excited after not walking alone for so long. Yes, I was excited that I was reaching my ultimate goal, but it was also really scary for me. I would actually cry sometimes, because I was so frightened. I remember thinking *I can't wait until walking alone isn't terrifying for me anymore!* Eventually walking became much easier and less scary, even though it took me a lot of practice for it to become faster and more stable.

When we began, I walked so slowly and deliberately because I had to in order to just stay balanced. I also had to swallow my pride a bit to use what I considered to be "old people things," like the walker and the canes. Still, I only saw the walker and canes as temporary and as a necessary way to get out of the wheelchair. I would have probably had a different attitude if I had had to accept them as permanent tools in my life. I also thought my single-point cane was special because it was my Grandpa Sieber's cane before he passed away. Later on, I used my Grandma Sieber's cane.

My physical therapy in LaCrosse, Wisconsin, was really great. My physical therapist, Kathy, was awesome and very dedicated to help me progress. I was a very young stroke patient. Most of the elderly patients were in the rehab room for knee and hip replacements. All of the older patients wondered why I was there because I was so young, but HIPAA privacy laws prevented the therapists from discussing why I was there, although I'm sure the other patients knew my story somehow.

The Gundersen Lutheran Hospital rehab center has a strong reputation in the area for stroke rehab. This knowledge was comforting because I didn't want to be an experiment. I was really ready to get better, and I wanted people with experience in stroke rehab who knew what I needed to do to make great progress. My parents liked Kathy too, the first day of therapy they told the therapist, "We read something claiming the treadmill is very important to stroke recovery, and we think this is necessary for Sara." "I think so, too," Kathy said, and she put me on the treadmill for five minutes every therapy session.

Initially, they put me into a harness, so that if I fell and the therapists couldn't grab me, the harness would prevent me from hitting the floor. I thought I would begin to walk without a cane while using the harness as well because it is safer, but Kathy thought it was better to start walking without anything because that would be more realistic for my goal. I remember Kathy first giving me a cane to try to walk with for the first time while the harness was around me, and that was terrifying, even with the harness. When you lack balance and don't know how to use a cane, it really is frightening!

When I stopped using the harness on the treadmill, I thought that was a big deal even though I couldn't see my progress. Any time the therapists became more trusting of me I knew it was a good sign. Kathy said I would need a brace on my left foot to prevent foot drag, but I had such bad memories from the foot drop boots that I was skeptical. I understood why I needed it, but I didn't want it to be painful. The purpose of the brace initially was to prevent toe drag. When I was on the treadmill, you could hear my left toe dragging when I walked. The bottom of my left shoe where this dragging occurred was always very smooth. This situation prompted Kathy to recommend a "toe up" brace, which is just a piece of fabric that wraps around your ankle and attaches to another part on the tongue of your shoe to keep your toe upright. I ended up borrowing one from Kathy to use in the therapy room.

However, shortly thereafter, Kathy recommended I get an ankle-foot orthosis (AFO), because in addition to keeping my toe up, I needed more ankle stability to prevent knee hyperextension, a problem for me on my left leg. It is actually quite a process to get a custom AFO. I had to visit an orthotist, who put some plaster on my leg to create a plaster cast for the AFO to get a custom fit. At least I was able to choose the color of the brace, which was fun. John, the orthotist, jokingly said that I could choose any color besides the Vikings' colors. (The Minnesota Vikings are a huge rival of Wisconsin's Green Bay Packers). I chose hot pink, which also made the brace very easy to spot. It took a couple weeks for the brace to be made.

After I received the brace, I also had to get it adjusted because it was bruising a bone on the inside of my foot. After that, however, it was comfortable, and I actually learned to like it because it provided the stability my foot was lacking. Kathy stressed that I should not become too dependent on the brace. After I had been wearing it for several months, Kathy then said that Dad should "wean" me off the brace. Dad's version of "wean" was to stop completely. I didn't wear the brace for a month, and then we noticed my ankle was becoming unstable again. We avoided any injury because I am very flexible, so my muscles could stretch enough not to be hurt. However, we both recognized the risk for a sprain or even a break, so I went back to wearing the brace again. I ended up wearing the AFO for years after receiving it, even while walking alone.

Also, with Kathy, I did something that surprised even me—bending over to pick something up. I had very poor balance; however, that motion of bending over to get something was okay for me. One day in therapy, Kathy purposely dropped something and asked me to pick it up.

Pretty confident I would be unsuccessful, I asked, "Are you sure?"

"Yes," Kathy said, pretty sure I would be successful.

"Okay, but I've never done this before," I warned her.

Not only did I doubt I had the balance to do what she had asked, I wasn't sure I had the leg strength yet to do it. However, therapists won't ask you to do something that they aren't somewhat confident you can do. So I bent down, picked up the object and straightened up with no problem. I was very pleasantly surprised I could do it, and I think it gave me a bit more confidence. I was really proud that I could do it.

I lacked confidence for a long time. Dad would say, "The greatest thing Sara is lacking is confidence." I completely agreed. However, confidence is something you can slowly gain. Since my balance was so bad, it was really hard to do so. In fact, I even had to slowly gain confidence in the other people who were holding my gait belt behind me. Dad or therapists would often say, "It's okay, I got you." However, I never felt fully confident unless I was hanging on to something. I tried to compare the feeling I had to walking on a tightrope. I thought that the feeling of potentially falling was like what you would imagine you'd feel if you were on a tightrope. It was similar to what I experienced, and also probably why I didn't enjoy walking. If you were walking on a tightrope and someone was holding on to a belt around your waist and saying, "I got you," I don't think anyone would feel confident in this situation. I felt bad for hurting others' feelings sometimes, and not being totally confident in whoever was with me, but I understood what I was feeling and that my feelings expressed my position.

One year post-stroke, as I previously described, I began to visit a nearby gym called the "Wellness Center." I had visited this gym prior to my stroke, so it was nice to go there now because I was familiar with the facility; however, this knowledge also caused me to feel more embarrassed because I knew the trainers remembered what I looked like before my stroke. Having to show what I looked like now after my stroke, and how limited I was in my ability, was pretty embarrassing for me. However,

I knew that weight training would be enormously beneficial, so once again, I swallowed my pride and visited on a regular basis. Fortunately, I ended up being a good example to the many visitors who came to the Wellness Center.

Later, in Wisconsin, we felt that more personal training could greatly improve my strength. So I began to work with a trainer from the Wellness Center. Every session we did something that was different from the session before. This trainer eventually left the Wellness Center, so Sam became my next trainer. I must admit, initially I was slightly apprehensive about switching trainers, but any fears I had were resolved immediately after working with Sam. I really enjoyed working him, and I don't think I could've been given a better trainer. I'm the same age as his sister, so I know Sam viewed me as a friend and really tried to do whatever he could to get me better.

I loved that Sam never made me feel like I was disabled or lacking in any way. He always treated me as an equal and completely overlooked my physical obstacles. Whereas my boyfriend Peter was super-critical of me after my stroke and only confirmed my insecurities, Sam really made me feel better about myself and helped me build my self-confidence even more. I was grateful to have Sam as my trainer. After Sam left the Wellness Center, my subsequent trainers at the Wellness Center were also all amazing and extremely helpful to me.

I also began to do reflexology. Reflexology is when the hands and mostly the feet are massaged, and their different pressure points correspond to different areas in the body. Bertha Johnson, who also taught at Westby High School with my dad, performs this therapy and she really wanted to work with me to see if it would help. I was excited too because I like and welcomed any natural therapies. It did work somewhat. I felt it helped me bring my foot muscles up. Bertha had other stroke clients too, and they mentioned similar benefits, and some of them even regained feeling! I was never lacking feeling, but I still found this point very interesting. My mom went too and she thought her sore hip definitely hurt less later in the day after her reflexology. As for me, I was more than ready to take any gains I could get.

When the insurance refused to pay for more therapy, I was very fortunate to be able to work with students and professors at the University of Wisconsin-LaCrosse (UWL) in their Exercise Program for Adults with Neurologic Disorders (EXPAND). I felt the PT girls, like the OT girls, truly embraced me and wanted me to recover as much as possible. I was approached one day to be the subject for a case study they wanted to conduct. I welcomed this opportunity and was happy they could take advantage of having me there. I felt I was a rarity, as I had a stroke so young and I also had so much drive to get better. However, they had to video record me at the start and finish to document my balance. I didn't like being recorded, or even photographed, so I signed a document saying that the video could only be used for research purposes. I even told the girls I didn't want to see it.

For the study, the girls performed many of the same exercises on me that I had performed in PT at various locations: sit-to-stand exercises, walking, squats, calf raises, bridges, etc. We did these activities twice a week during our sessions. In the end, I was happy to see that I had improved in all areas. After the girls also assured me I had improved, I watched the video. Any doubt that I wasn't progressing was put to rest upon witnessing my video. I undeniably saw a big difference in my balance and my brain rewiring. I made sure both my parents watched the video too. I remember in California that I was so embarrassed to do any therapy in front of my parents that I would ask to have the curtains drawn around the mat tables and ask not to walk where my parents were because I was so ashamed of what I couldn't do. However, so much time had passed now that I knew that they were fully on this journey with me and they deserved to witness the video as much as I did. They were very proud of me too.

I was later introduced to a therapeutic swimming program at UWL that was supervised by Dr. Emmanuel (Manny) Felix. I typically worked with students in the pool, and Manny would supervise. I had liked being in the water before for therapy, as it was very comforting to swim again. I was not afraid to fall when I was in the water and often thought how nice it would be to have that same balance out of the water. I was impressed how easily I could swim despite my disability. Of course I was always supervised, but even when I wasn't, I was confident I wouldn't drown because I could tread water just fine and stay afloat.

About five years post-stroke, I decided to attend one-on-one yoga sessions with Christine Saudek. She is not only an incredibly talented and well-known yoga instructor, but also a former physical therapist. That made her the perfect person to work with me. Before the stroke, I was definitely one of those people who doubted yoga was exercise. It just seemed like stretching. However, yoga soon became my most challenging activity, hands down. Chris really challenged me, and I was exhausted after our sessions, much more so than after all of the other therapies.

Yoga was very effective at strengthening my body, among other things. Chris was very skilled at identifying muscle imbalances and trying to help me correct them with yoga activities. Since I didn't know Chris as anything but my yoga instructor, I asked one of her students, Carol Anne Kemen to describe her in more detail for me. She says:

> she has been enthusiastically teaching yoga for over thirty years now, and has traveled to Pune, India many times to study directly with the yoga master B.K.S. Iyengar, his daughter Geeta, and his son Prashant. She is a totally devoted practitioner of Iyengar Yoga, and to her, yoga is a way of life, as she strives to live in a way that is guided by the philosophy of yoga as set out in the ancient text of The Yoga Sutras. She considers herself to always be a student of yoga, challenging herself to improve and grow through yogic practices. She has conducted yoga teacher study groups for many years in Madison and LaCrosse, Wisconsin, and has mentored and challenged a plethora of teachers to become their best selves, thereby spreading the gift of yoga throughout the US and beyond. Chris travels around the US, and to Canada, to teach workshops, and is well respected as a Senior Teacher within the world-wide Iyengar Yoga Community.

Many times Chris would ask me to do something that I thought was impossible for me to do, and then I could actually do it, which was wonderful for me to see. She was very challenging, in the best way possible. Unlike all the other therapies, after a little more than a year in yoga, I could actually notice my balance getting better, especially my standing balance. I also noticed myself doing certain tasks like washing the dishes or brushing my teeth without leaning against the counter in front of me. I think all my therapies actually combined to help me achieve this change, but I especially attribute that success to yoga. I would credit my one-on-one yoga sessions as being the most beneficial therapy for me in my entire rehab. I think the individual sessions were key and delivered the individual attention and assistance I needed. Previously I had tried a yoga video at home by myself, but I can now say it was worthless compared to my individual lessons.

Yoga with Chris Saudek

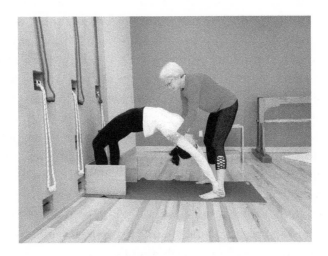

Since I had such good results with yoga over the course of one semester at UWL, one of the students working with me named Laura asked if I would be interested in learning Tai Chi. I immediately agreed. I didn't know anything about Tai Chi, but in a nutshell, I would describe it as standing weight shift motions, while simultaneously using your arms to do movements. This is my description as a non-Tai Chi expert. It is, of course, much more. Actually, I was pleasantly surprised at how much coordination it involves for the arms too. I felt it was helpful for both of my biggest deficits from my stroke that I was working so hard to overcome: balance and coordination. Laura helped me with some of the exercises that we did in therapy, and when the semester ended, she gave me a YouTube video to help me with the exercises in the future. That video can be seen at https://www.youtube.com/watch?v=PNtWqDxwwMg

My Tai Chi practice was very informal, and although this video says eight minutes, it took me between twenty to twenty-five minutes to complete it. That is due to the fact that the video's instructor only demonstrates a few repetitions, whereas I did up to ten. It also took me longer to switch Tai Chi positions because of my mobility issues. When I did the work at home independently, I found the perfect place to do it to avoid falls—in front of my bed and in between a doorway with the door opening in on my right (stronger) side. Then I could use the door to adjust my balance, which I often did. My walker was on my left side, so I had something on all sides of me protecting me. I knew my arms would brace me if I fell forward. Tai Chi was a great activity to heal my balance and coordination. It also gave me more confidence because I could do it independently!

Several months after I began yoga, I re-evaluated my cardio-vascular fitness. As I previously mentioned, my cardiovascular fitness was excellent prior to my stroke, and I wanted to get that back. However, I also wanted to focus on high intensity interval training (HIIT) rather than the long constant cardio routine I did before the stroke. This decision was based on information I'd read in various fitness magazines saying that HIIT training for a fraction of the time can help one achieve similar, if not better, results than a single intensity, long workout. Good results in less time sounded really great to me! I thought that ten minutes seemed like a good time span for my goal, which according to HIIT would also give me a better workout than a much longer, constant-intensity workout.

With HIIT, as the name suggests, you do a series of high intensity intervals, followed by resting intervals. For the high intensity part, you go as hard as you can, and then recover and repeat this same sequence several times. Of course, I would recommend consulting a doctor and a personal trainer to figure out what works best for you.

My first choice was to get an elliptical machine since that's what I used pre-stroke, but after considering the nature of the high intensity intervals, I decided against it because I knew my quality would be too poor to perform a HIIT workout with this machine. However, we had a stationary bike, so I decided to use it because I was seated, and therefore, I could perform the intervals more easily and well.

I would wake up and do this workout first thing in the morning. I also think it's a better idea to start at a lower number, say five minutes, and add a minute each week to build up to more minutes. So please consult your doctor first. I was pleasantly surprised that I could even perform this program and without much difficulty. After a handful of years not doing much related to cardio, I was so happy to get my cardiovascular endurance back again. Better yet, it made my other activities easier too. I used to feel so exhausted after my yoga session, but after I intro-duced cardio back into my daily routine, yoga was not leaving me so depleted. I think it was very important for me to focus on my cardiovascular fitness in order to gain more endurance. This extra endurance helped me in all my other therapies.

My favorite therapy was massage therapy. Occasionally, I would visit my massage therapist, Sam, for a one hour full body massage. Before the stroke, I rarely would have treated myself to a massage appointment. However, post-stroke I was working so hard with many different therapies, that I felt my massage therapy appointments were well deserved, and also a great and enjoyable way to send brain to body messages.

One of my favorite responses to my therapists around this time was using my stroke as an excuse for everything that I did incorrectly. Often, therapists asked me, "Why are you doing that?" "I had a stroke," I would reply. I meant it as kind of a smart-ass answer to tease them, but it was an accurate answer as well. I don't think they were expecting any response, rather just thinking aloud, but I still often answered this way. I did the same outside of therapy too. Because it was the therapists' thoughts to themselves, I often got laughs from them because they weren't expecting a response. However, since my family heard that response from me all the time, they got tired of hearing it.

Therapy is talked about like it is the "magic cure" after a stroke, but I don't think therapy is "magic." However, I do think it's very necessary. When I was coming to terms with what had happened to me, I asked everyone how to get better, and everyone said "therapy." I agree, but I also think time should be emphasized too. I know that's a frustrating thought because you can't control time, but that is what helped in my case. However, I also know that when our insurance ran out, everyone was afraid my progress would regress too. I didn't regress, but only because of the hours of home therapy I did and a lot of time. I wasn't concerned about backsliding because I knew I had a lot of personal motivation and a good home routine, and those are not entirely common or available for everybody. You can get around insurance with a good home routine. However, I can't stress enough that one's self-motivation and personal determination and dedication is essential to do so.

I noticed that therapists like having the reputation of being mean. Some people will say that therapists assume that if a patient calls them mean, that means he or she is a good therapist. I never believed this. I never met a therapist I didn't like or one that I thought was "mean." In fact, I often sought out the "mean" therapists to see if they really were mean but they never were. I knew they wanted to get me better, and I always appreciated that support.

As in OT, "reaching" was an issue in PT. Again, I would reach for a counter or a railing because these physical things were much more stable than I was. I always wanted to grab on to things to help my balance. I knew that this act was not helping my balance, but I still wanted to constantly grab for things because I wanted to feel safe. I hated it when in therapy we would use the parallel bars, and the therapist would say, "Only use the bars if you need them!" I always wanted to use them, and I felt I needed to use them. The same thing happened at home when I first began walking without an assistive device. We would walk around the counters and I was told to use the counters "only if needed," but I always wanted them for my own sense of security.

It was actually easier, although initially scarier, to walk in the open and out of arms reach of anything because the temptation to reach for something was not there. I still used anything I could for more stability input. I would often "hit Dad in the gut" with my elbow, or even hit the back of my hand at whoever was walking behind me. This contact would give me the input I wanted and a sense of relief that someone was nearby to catch me if needed. If I was walking with a cane, I would lean it up against a wall for extra stability. Mom called this "cheating." However in my own defense, it really is hard to balance with a cane!

Discussing physical input as it related to my gait, the gait belt is also important to mention here. A gait belt is a belt that wraps around the waist of people who have balance issues, so that individual can easily be rebalanced by someone else. I had to wear one every day. It was really big around the waist, so the extra length that hung behind me is called "the tail" because that's what it resembles. Kathy told my parents to hold the tail because the tail does not give as much input. She was right too. I could definitely tell the difference, and I found it was much harder to walk when someone just held the tail.

Dad wanted to have a "wheelchair burning party" to symbolize my freedom from it, but Mom said we could not do that because the wheelchair was a rental from the insurance company, so instead, we shifted our focus to a "gait belt burning party." We didn't actually end up burning it because we didn't have an appropriate place to do so. However, we were very happy when I stopped wearing and needing it. I had worn it for several years I had a love-hate relationship with the gait belt. We all hated that I needed it, but we loved the belt when I stumbled because it was so much easier to adjust my balance using it. Sometimes it seemed like Dad caught me in mid-air with the gait belt to prevent me from hitting the floor.

Overall, PT played a very large part in my recovery. Walking was my main goal. I practiced so hard and waited so long to get there. I thought I'll never take walking for granted because I've had to work so hard to get this back again. I also felt very thankful that I was lucky enough to have the ability to graduate at last from the wheelchair. I knew walking was essential to reaching my goal of resuming my former life, and also that that new life would require a lot of balance in many ways.

CHAPTER 21

Speech Therapy

SPEECH WAS MY third therapy and probably my favorite. I have always had an interest in languages, so I had that in common with my speech therapists. I was very grateful not to have suffered from aphasia as a result of my stroke. That is when you lose your vocabulary, your ability to communicate, and your concept of language in general. My stroke occurred more on the right hemisphere of my brain, giving me more weakness on the left side of my body. Language centers are typically located in the left hemisphere of the brain. Jen, who I met at the Topanga Terrace rehab center, had a stroke in her left hemisphere, and she experienced aphasia. She said it took an awfully long time for her to regain her vocabulary and speak, read and write again. Fortunately, I did not have these problems. While I suffered many other physical limitations, I was very thankful that I always kept all my cognitive and language skills, even though I was unable to communicate verbally for months. I remember discussing aphasia in a phonology class when I was an undergraduate, so I knew about aphasia, but I certainly never would have thought that it would have hit so close to home and in my twenties no less!

Even though I didn't experience aphasia, I did have my own speech issues. I was initially diagnosed with "ataxic dysarthria." Those around me the most complained that I spoke too quickly and too quietly. After I finally regained my voice, we realized that the stroke had caused me to speak very quickly and repeat what I said three times. I simply could not control my rate of speech nor increase my volume. I remember talking one time and Dad asking me sarcastically "Can you talk any faster?" and I thought, *No, actually, I can't.* Dad doesn't have the world's greatest hearing. So, since we worked together daily, it was good speech practice for me because I had to speak clearly and loudly enough for him to hear me, or he would ask me to repeat myself. That was often.

My communication progress was slow. I began by not being able to speak at all, so I had to communicate at first with eye blinks to answer "yes" or "no" questions. As you can imagine, this kind of communication was very inconsistent and difficult. Then when I started to move my right hand, Patti in PT at Topanga Terrace suggested that I signal thumbs up for "yes" and thumbs down for "no." To tease me, my Dad would then ask me "Sara, can I change the TV channel to the golf channel?" I would hide my thumb with my fingers as if to say *No way!*

One weekend, much later in my recovery, I went to Fond du Lac, Wisconsin, with my Dad to visit Lynda, his girlfriend. We were all sitting in her living room and Dad had the golf channel on, so jokingly I said "Hey Dad!" then I held up my thumb hidden with my fingers, so he knew he should change the channel. Everyone was very happy that I could do thumbs up or thumbs down because it was easier to communicate with me. Still, it was difficult for me to convey any complex thoughts without speech. I simply lived in a world of "yes" or "no" for months. I learned that almost anything can be phrased into a "yes" or "no" question, but I could not ask questions. Peter would visit after work and ask, "Sara how is your body temperature? Are you too hot? Are you too cold?" I always appreciated this question because sometimes I did want to adjust my temperature, and it could be easily remedied.

Around this time, I was also offered an alphabet board to spell things out by pointing, which I loved and I would have liked sooner. I would always think in advance what I would spell out the next time I was offered the board. Since I had my vocabulary intact and I could use my right hand enough, the alphabet board became a very useful tool. One of the first things I wrote out to my parents was "I'm so sorry" because I felt really bad that they had needed to leave their own lives to be with me. I also repeatedly tried to spell out "wake me up now" because I wanted to be awakened from my nightmare very badly. Mom would say, "Sara, you're not sleeping!" But I was sure I had to be sleeping because everything was so weird to me. Trapped in a hospital bed, not being able to move or talk made no sense to me. Eventually, after several months, I got some movement back in my neck, and I could slightly nod my head "yes" or slightly shake it for "no." That felt like a huge step forward in communication. Again, during this time, I was not making any sounds or even attempting to speak. I suppose my brain had yet to make the right physical connections to allow me to communicate using my voice.

After months, I could mouth words, but it was rare that anyone could understand me because I was not making any definitive sounds. I remember my mom saying, "I wish I could read lips!" I remember thinking that if I could communicate one thing a day that would be a victory in my book. I rarely succeeded at it, however. When I started mouthing words, I attempted to mouth "wake me," but no one could get it. Mom could get the "me" part, because the /m/ is bilabial, so "me" is easier for someone to guess. My linguistics training helped me because I was able to analyze what I was mouthing. I wondered why people couldn't understand "wake me." I thought the /w/ and /m/ are bilabial, but the /k/ sound is velar which is produced in the back of your mouth and would be nearly impossible to understand. However, I couldn't think of another way to better communicate my message.

I was desperately trying to end the dream, my nightmare, trying anything I could, so I thought maybe by communicating my message of "wake me" it would actually end. It didn't, and not being able to speak did produce some very terrifying moments for me. Was I going to live in a world where I could not communicate? That thought was very isolating and scary. I remember one time I was trying to mouth "wake me up" and Mom caught the /w/ and said "Sara, are you trying to say 'what'?" That's not what I was saying since "wake" was my intent, but I was so confused, that I just nodded my head "yes," hoping for more explanation. Mom then told me about the stroke and my whole family coming to visit me, but I did not believe any of it. I was young and healthy and nothing in my lifestyle had ever resembled anything even close to being a health risk.

I remember one night I awoke in my bed at Topanga Terrace. The foot drop boots were on my feet and causing me a lot of pain. I was able to push the nurse button, but I was unable to communicate my message. I tried to think of any way that I could communicate how much I hated the boots because I felt my life would be improved so much if I did not have to wear them. I even thought of spelling out "no boots please" on the alphabet board. However, I was also convinced I was trapped in a nightmare, and if I could make that nightmare end, the boots and everything else that terrified me would be gone too. Later, my mom wrote out phrases on a sheet of paper, such as "I'm thirsty," "I'm cold" etc. and gave these to the nurses for me to read and point to as I needed to communicate what I needed. I thought it was a great idea, and I definitely could have used that list much earlier.

Although I could not speak, I had some movement in my right hand, so my mom told me to hold up two fingers to signal that I wanted two cookies and a glass of milk. My parents referred to this communication as the "two cookie salute." Ice cream and cookies soaked in milk were among the first things I ate after the stroke. Very unhealthy, I know, but after being fed through a tube for three months, I did not care. Also, I thought I was in a dream all this time, so I did not think the calories really counted anyway when I eventually woke up. I was very upset when I realized that was not the case. Sometimes I would also do the "two-cookie salute" just for the glass of milk because I was so thirsty. When my Grandma Anderson visited in the summer, she brought along some of her sugar cookies, and they are legendary in my family. However, my speech therapist at the time said they were "too crumbly" for me to eat, so I could not have them because they could be too difficult for me to swallow correctly. I was really disappointed to say the very least.

After I could mouth words, I began to slightly whisper. While whispering certainly was not ideal, I was very happy to whisper because at least I could communicate a bit and get my point across. Finally, I could communicate more than "yes" or "no." Plus, I still had my language, which I was so very thankful I hadn't lost. However, the linguist inside me also thought, "Why can't I voice consonants?" Then after a few weeks of working on sounds, my whispering became a bit more audible. Everyone had to lean close to hear me, but I was actually "talking." After several more months, my volume got better bit by bit. Finally I was regaining my voice. My pitch however was a little lower, and we compared it to the voicemail recording on my cell phone that I had made before the stroke. It was the only voice recording I had, but it was very useful because all my speech therapists wanted to hear my voice before the stroke to have a precise reference point. Since I now spoke much quieter, many of the therapists suggested a voice amplifier, which I declined. It was "stroke related." As long as I could be understood, I did not want any gadget to help me. I wanted to see how much of my voice would come back naturally.

I had many wonderful speech therapists who worked with me throughout my recovery. The first was Padi from Topanga Terrace. My parents nicknamed her "Ice Cream Padi." This nickname was to distinguish her from my physical therapist, also named Patti, different spelling, but same pronunciation. Padi began every therapy session by feeding me ice cream, saying it would lubricate my vocal cords to facilitate my speaking. I thought this was kind of silly, but I enjoyed it, and there were not many things I enjoyed in those days. Padi was actually the most likely therapist to get neck movement from me, depending on where she positioned the spoonful of ice cream. Often during our speech sessions, Padi would say, "Sara, just open your mouth and say 'ahhhh'." I would open my mouth, but no sound would come out. Another time, I remember my task was simply to blow bubbles, but I couldn't, a clear indication of how weak my diaphragm was then.

Another area that the therapists supervised during speech therapy was swallowing to make sure I was not at risk for choking. As a result, Padi scheduled me for a "swallow study" to test how well I could handle different consistencies of liquids. For this study, I had to go to another hospital where they took an x-ray of my neck and chest before and after the test to make sure I had not aspirated anything into my lungs. They had me swallow various consistencies from yogurt-like to honey-like. I passed the test, so I was especially upset when Padi later vetoed Grandma's cookies. Regardless, we were all very excited that I had passed the swallow study because it was a sign that I was healing, and soon I would hopefully be getting rid of the G-tube and start eating normal food again.

My passing that test also gave my mom even more motivation to petition for removing the trach from my throat. In addition to how awful the trach tube looked going into my throat, she felt it was hindering my progress with breathing, swallowing and speaking. So she wanted it out as soon as possible. When I was with Padi, the biggest goal for me was to make any sounds at all. I remember Padi telling my mom "Sharon, you should be hired because you're so helpful!" Mom was also doing all she could to help me formulate sounds and words. Padi was my speech therapist when I was first able to talk again. She was very kind to my parents and me. I was very sad that I had to leave Padi when I left Topanga for Northridge.

Mimi was my speech therapist at Northridge Hospital. Our first session was evaluative, as Mimi wanted to see how well I could chew and swallow food. She had me chew and swallow a dried apricot, which she thought I had some difficulty doing. I pleaded with Mimi not to limit my food choices, because I remembered the fiasco when Padi rejected Grandma Anderson's cookies and I did not want anything like that to happen again. Mimi told me, "I will write down that you will need vegetable broth with every meal with the intention that you will soak your food in it, so it is easier to swallow." So every day the broth came, and of course I never used it. I was confident now that I could chew and swallow food properly. However, she just had to do something because she thought I had difficulty with the apricot.

Mimi was also the leader of my "pet therapy." To try to get out of pet therapy, I told Mimi that I did not want to go because "I don't like Nick," the poodle. But really, I just did not want to be in a room with other patients and talking about ourselves due to my insecurities. Nick was the poodle that came along for pet therapy. Mimi thought it was very important for me to be part of a small group and practice speaking out loud because of my career in teaching, so I spoke very quietly. Mimi was also the leader of a lunch group that sat together and talked. She told me I had to join one or the other. I chose pet therapy because I actually did like Nick and the pet therapy, and I also ended up enjoying the people in the group as well. The poodle was a great friend because animals automatically are your friend with no judgment so I didn't have to feel insecure around Nick. I suppose that group was really my first step in socializing with others outside of my family. I was just so embarrassed about my physical limitations that I felt insecure being around all others, but I slowly made some inroads and progressed in the group.

My speech therapist in Wisconsin was Vicki. Vicki and I are alike in many ways. We are both pescatarian, we both love languages, and we both love animals. Vicki definitely was an advocate for me to get my vocal cords looked at via a closer examination. This procedure had never been done on me before, even though I was intubated from the tracheotomy that had been performed on me. Vicki was doubtful there had been any damage done to my vocal cords, but we wanted to rule it out as a possibility for why I was not able to produce much volume.

Vicki scheduled an appointment for me with Dr. Hartman to closely look at my vocal cords. For this appointment Dr. Hartman put a metal bar with a camera at the back of my mouth to look down my throat. Then he told me to say some vowel sounds. The camera then displayed on the computer what my vocal cords were doing. I thought this process was so cool because I had never seen vocal cords before even though I had studied phonology and taught English pronunciation. I had also always thought it was interesting how we produce sounds. Vicki came to this appointment with me because she was very curious about what was going on with my vocal cords. After this procedure, it was determined that no harm was done to my vocal cords, but they were not adducting, or closing properly whenever I spoke. Because of this inadequate adducting, it made my voice sound kind of breathy when I spoke.

At home, I would practice reading articles out loud each day. That way I could practice hearing myself—both my clarity and my speech rate. It was important for me to slow down my speech in order to speak clearer, and project my voice more in order to be more audible. I had to retrain myself in both breathing and speaking by pausing at commas, periods, and paragraph breaks. This tactic also helped me slow my speech down to a more normal rate, so people could understand me better. My speech deficits were something I also tried to improve on daily through physical exercises that built my diaphragm, as well as general daily conversation and reading aloud.

Speech, PT, and OT were my three regular forms of therapy. I enjoyed my speech therapy most because I love language skills. Not being able to speak for months left me with some terrible memories. I was truly relieved to finally find my voice again, even though I had deficits still to overcome.

CHAPTER 22

Living Back in God's Country

ALWAYS ENVISIONED California to be my last chapter of my journal because that's where my life was before the stroke. However, I went through a break-up with Peter, so my plans changed. Many people assumed I'd take off again as soon as I could since I'd lived in so many faraway places previously. However, at this point in my life and after all I'd been through, sticking close to home sounded great to me. I could watch my nephews and nieces grow up and are close to family again. I don't think I ever would have guessed I'd end up living in the same small town where I grew up, but it didn't sound like a bad option now. I love Wisconsin. Home is where the heart is, and there is a lot to be said for that, Wisconsin winters and all.

Final thoughts on an unexpected journey

I have some final words I want to give to stroke survivors: You need to find your own motivation to help you get through this ordeal. If you can't do it for yourself, do it for someone else: your family, friends, spouse, whoever! It's very important to identify exactly what motivates you because stroke recovery is very repetitive and monotonous. You really have to find your own motivation to stay persistent and recover. If you do embrace rehab, however, the nagging stops! Naggers, you need to let up once you see an effort being made! Another piece of advice is: beat a plateau by changing your routine. I would notice a plateau appear occasionally when I was testing my OT scores monthly. Then, I would change whatever OT exercises I was doing, so the next month I could continue to see progress. I would also completely change my therapy occasionally to try to avoid any plateau, and that seemed to work better. Finally, when hearing a story like mine, it's always so easy to think, *Glad it wasn't me!* This is a very natural reaction! However, my advice to you is to protect yourself and others!

Use my story as a lesson and learn from it! Tell my story to everyone you know and spread the details about the dangers of contra-indicated medications. To repeat, in my case, I was using a combined estrogen and progesterone birth control pill while experiencing migraines with aura, but there are many more contra-indications! Again, progesterone-only birth control is the "safest." Please double check all your medications and vitamins for those contra-indications and others that doctors may have failed to point out to you.